365 Custom Cardio Fitness Workouts

365 Custom Cardio Fitness Workouts

SIMPLE EFFECTIVE CARDIO ROUTINES
FOR ALL LEVELS OF FITNESS

Justin A. Vida, MBA

ISBN: 1512046132
ISBN 13: 9781512046137
Library of Congress Control Number: 2015907593
CreateSpace Independent Publishing Platform
North Charleston, South Carolina

To my family, who always believes
in me and shows endless support.
For my parents, who gave me
all I ever needed and more
than I could ever want.

Remember – all things are possible
for those who believe.

OBSERVATION

I once was speaking with a person who had been doing cardiovascular training for one to two hours a day, five days a week for five years, and this person did not lose a single pound. She was performing the same or similar workouts every day. While structure and accountability are important, her routine had no variety. The key to getting results is tricking the muscles, that is, keeping them guessing as to which exercises they will have to perform. In addition, the woman was not committed to eating healthy foods, which limited her capacity for results. She could not lose weight and inches because she lacked variety in her routine and nutrition in her diet. Having been in the fitness industry for over fifteen years, I have talked with thousands of clients and gym members. I have realized that most of them do not know how to effectively execute cardiovascular training to burn fat.

Use the guidance in this book to ensure that your body draws its fuel from fat cells and that you keep your heart rate in your personal fat-burning zone. As a person becomes more fit, his or her heart becomes more efficient at pumping blood to the rest of the body. Cardiovascular workouts are very important contributors to this process. In addition, I strongly recommend a strength-training program along with a focused nutrition plan to maximize results. Teach your body to become an efficient fat burner, not a fat storer. You may have one hundred reasons why you can't test your limits, but this book will help you create a life you deserve. In addition, it will help you:

1. Push your body
2. Expand your limits
3. Discover and gain strength
4. Create optimal change

It will also guide you on how far to go and how far not to go. Exercise can actually be enjoyable, but you should never compare yourself to anyone else. In addition, you should never begin an exercise program without consulting your medical doctor first.

Don't be overwhelmed by the thought of an "entire cardiovascular session"; this book will break it down for you minute by minute. It uses patterns and numerical data to create a routine that is easy to follow and effective. There is a light at the end of the tunnel.

The Benefits of Cardiovascular Training

What will I notice when I begin to exercise?

Aerobic training increases your lung capacity and forces your heart to pump more blood to your body, which strengthens the heart. In addition, weight loss boosts the fat-burning metabolism; allows more rest on fewer hours of sleep; slows bone loss; provides relief to the joints; can help alleviate depression; decreases the risk of heart disease and cancer; can help reduce stress, anxiety, and lethargy; decreases body fat; and strengthens the heart and lungs.

Benefits of regular cardio training:

- Increased endurance levels
- Weight loss
- Reduction of inches, typically around the waist and hips
- Better-fitting clothes
- Heightened energy levels
- Improved sleep
- Increased flexibility
- Decreased body fat
- Lessened chance of heart disease
- Lower cholesterol levels
- Increased bone density

How often should I do cardio training?

Cardio training should be done a minimum of three times per week to stay fairly fit and to keep your heart healthy. If this is your goal, then I would recommend cardio training three or four days per week.

If you want to burn more calories and your goal is to lose weight and inches, then I would recommend cardio training five or six times per week. But you must remember to create balance in your routine. In addition to your cardio session, you must complete resistance training two or three days per week, and you must stay focused on your nutrition plan.

Again, the universal goal is to infuse variety into your routine. This book will give you variety because every single workout is different!

What do I need to exercise?

These items are necessary for a good workout:

- This book
- A writing utensil (or e-reader)
- Sneakers
- Gym clothes
- A water bottle
- A smile
- A positive, "never quit" attitude

These items are not necessary, but are helpful:

- A watch (with heart rate monitoring capability; I would recommend Polar)
- A towel

Consult your physician before exercising.

Determining Your Workout Level

What is a Target-Heart-Rate zone?

Below you will have three options to determine the appropriate work-out level for you. Choose the option that you prefer.

Option 1: The heart rate watch
Personally I would recommend a Polar heart rate watch and monitor. They are very durable and accurate (and they come in all different colors). Wearing a heart-rate monitor is the easiest and most accurate way of measuring your resting heart rate (RHR). However, below is an illustration that shows you how to calculate it.

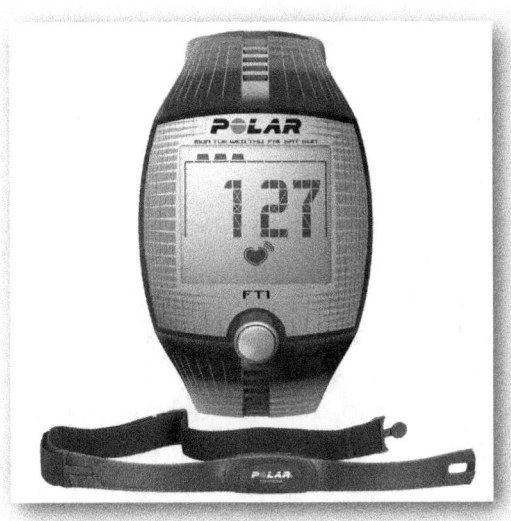

Option 2: The heart rate chart
Use the chart below to locate the specific numbers in which you should train to have the most effective cardio workout.

TRAINING HEART RATE ZONES

189	**180**	171	162	153	144	135	126	117	
168	**160**	152	144	136	128	120	112	104	
147	**140**	133	126	119	112	105	98	91	
126	**120**	114	108	102	96	90	84	78	
105	**100**	95	90	85	80	75	70	65	
10	**20**	**30**	**40**	**50**	**60**	**70**	**80**	**90**	

HEART RATE (vertical axis)

ANAEROBIC ZONE 80% – 90%
AEROBIC ZONE 70% – 80%
WEIGHT CONTROL ZONE 60% – 70%
FAT-BURNING ZONE 50% – 60%

AGE

Option 3: The Karvonen Formula, the most scientific option
This is a mathematical formula that helps you determine your target-heart-rate (HR) training zone. The formula plots maximum and resting heart rates against desired training intensities to get target-heart rates for each combination. Staying within the range you choose will help you work most effectively—and burn fat during your cardio workouts.

When resting, the number of heartbeats per minute slows down. To find out what your most accurate target-heart-rate should be while exercising, you will need to determine your resting heart rate (RHR). The best time to check your resting rate is just before you get up in the morning after a good night's sleep. Take the average of two or three mornings' readings for greater accuracy.

Finding your RHR:

https://fitnessmodule.files.wordpress.com/2010/03/picture2.png

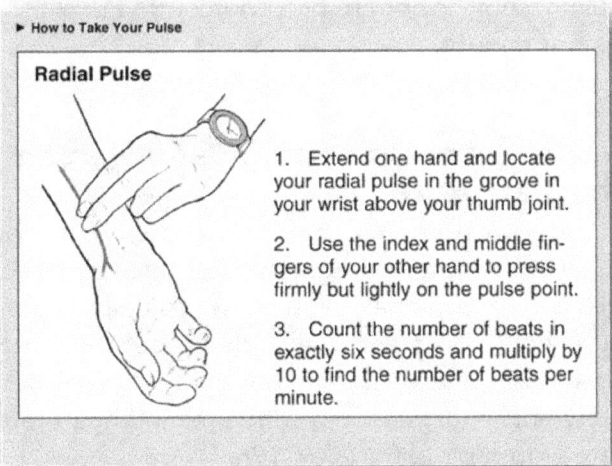

▶ How to Take Your Pulse

Radial Pulse

1. Extend one hand and locate your radial pulse in the groove in your wrist above your thumb joint.

2. Use the index and middle fingers of your other hand to press firmly but lightly on the pulse point.

3. Count the number of beats in exactly six seconds and multiply by 10 to find the number of beats per minute.

Finding your Target-Heart-Rate zone (60–70 percent of your maximum HR):

This zone provides the same benefits as the healthy heart zone, but it is more intense and burns more total calories. The formula to determine your maximum HR is:

220 – your age = your maximum HR (HR max).

To find your Target-Heart-Rate zone, do the following:

1. Subtract your resting heart rate (RHR) from your HR max.
2. Calculate lower limit (60 percent): multiply by 0.6 and add your RHR.
3. Calculate upper limit (70 percent): multiply by 0.7 and add your RHR.

For example, if you are twenty-four years old with a resting heart rate of 78, you would use the following method to calculate your max heart rate:

220 – 24 = 196.

1. Subtract RHR from HR max: 196 – 78 = 118.

2. Calculate your lower limit (60 percent): 118 x 0.6 + 78 = 149 beats per minute.
3. Calculate your upper limit (70 percent): 118 x 0.7 + 78 = 160 beats per minute.

Finding your Warm-Up zone (50–60 Percent of the Maximum Heart Rate):

This zone is the lowest-impact zone and probably the best zone for people just starting a fitness program. It can also be used as a warm-up for exercisers. This zone has been shown to help decrease body fat, blood pressure, and cholesterol. It also decreases the risk of degenerative diseases and has a low risk of injury.

If you are twenty-four years old with a resting heart rate of 78, your max heart rate would be 220 – 24 = 196.

1. RHR from HR max: 196 – 78 = 118.
2. Calculate your lower limit (50 percent): 118 x 0.5 + 78 = 137 beats per minute.
3. Calculate your upper limit (60 percent): 118 x 0.6 + 78 = 149 beats per minute.

Finding your Aerobic zone (endurance training; 70–80 Percent of Maximum Heart Rate):

The aerobic zone will improve your cardiovascular and respiratory system as well as increase your aerobic capacity and the strength of your heart. This is the preferred zone if you are training for an endurance event.

If you are twenty-four years old with a resting heart rate of 78, your max heart rate would be 220 – 24 = 196.

1. Subtract RHR from HR max: 196 – 78 = 118.
2. Calculate your upper limit (70 percent): 118 x 0.7 + 78 = 160 beats per minute.
3. Calculate your upper limit (80 percent): 118 x 0.8 + 78 = 172 beats per minute.

CARDIOVASCULAR TRAINING TIPS

When you step onto your piece of cardio equipment, select the manual or quick-start option. If asked, input your personal data (height, weight, etc.), and then begin the session.

Avoid doing cardio exercises before bedtime. You may have difficulty sleeping due to the fact that the energy level of the body will stay high for some time.

If you are undergoing weight training, too, complete your cardio exercises right after it, not before. If your heart rate begins to climb out of your zone, slow down. If you are below your allotted target-heart-rate zone, increase the speed, revolutions per minute, or resistance level.

What should I eat and drink?

It is best to eat a snack 60 to 90 minutes before doing the cardio exercises. This snack should include a complex carbohydrate and a protein. Do not start training on an empty stomach, and avoid indulging in large meals before exercise. This will not help achieve the proper momentum when you train.

Suggested Pre-Workout Foods:

- Banana
- Multigrain bar/crackers

- Oatmeal
- Apple
- Sweet potato
- Peanut butter
- Greek yogurt
- Smoothie
- Berries
- Eggs
- English muffin
- Quinoa
- Dried fruit
- Veggie omelet

Suggested Post-Workout Foods:

- Protein bar/shake
- Trail mix
- Tuna
- Bagel and egg whites
- Apples and cheese
- Cottage cheese
- Rice cakes and peanut butter
- Pita and hummus
- Chicken and veggies
- Fish
- Chocolate milk
- Wraps
- Fruit salad

Hydrate, hydrate, hydrate!

Drink a lot of water. Make sure you drink 8 to 14 ounces of water, 30 to 60 minutes prior to exercising. During exercise, sip water as needed. Remember that your body is going to be sweating, which can cause dehydration. Post workout, drink a minimum of 12 to 18 ounces of water to help rehydrate. Remember, everyone is different, and what works for one person might not work for you.

Keep a journal to help you:

- Track your progress
- See the positive changes
- Recognize progress toward goals
- Identify success
- Break through plateaus
- Find motivation and get positive feedback
- Release your thoughts and feelings
- Cleanse the mind and soul

Be consistent, and stick with it once you start training. This is the only way your cardiovascular training will benefit you.

Cardio Equipment and Substitutes

If there is no level, speed, or incline indicated, you have the freedom to pick the setting that keeps you in your target-heart-rate zone.

Machines:

Treadmill

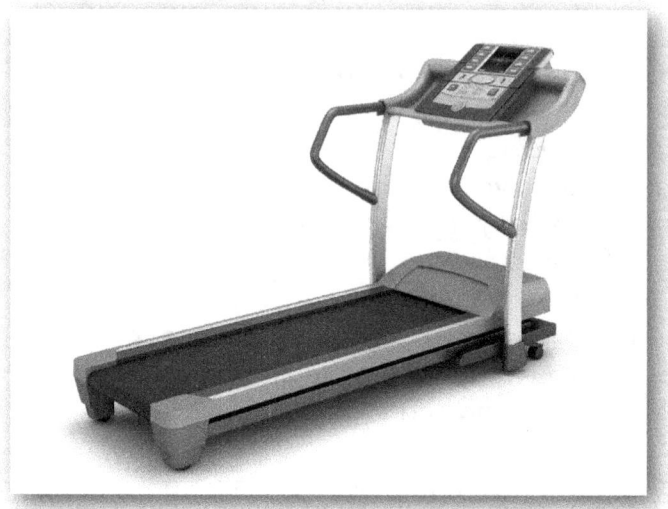

Elliptical

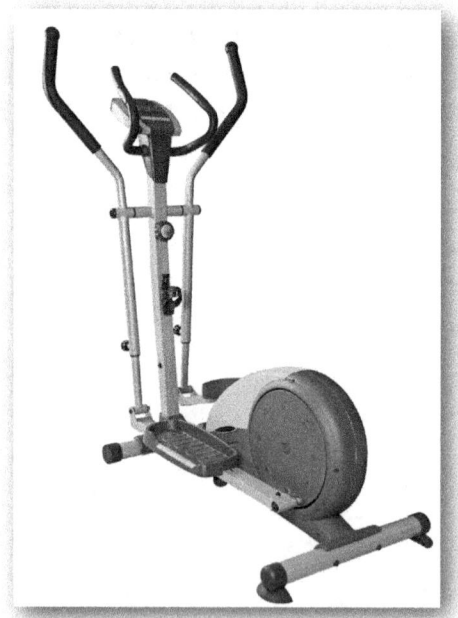

Cybex arc trainer

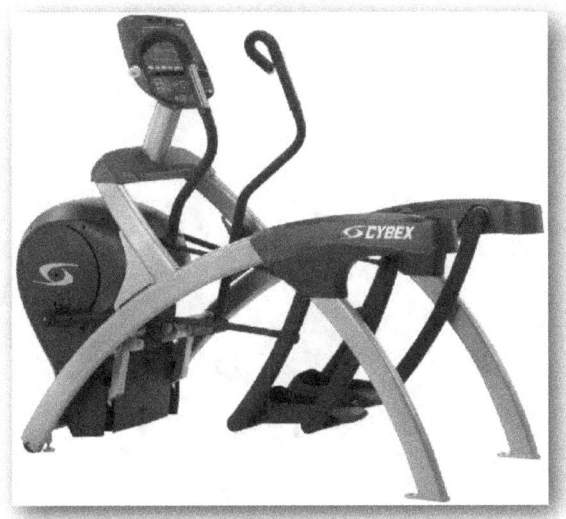

http://www.cybexintl.com/

Recumbent bike

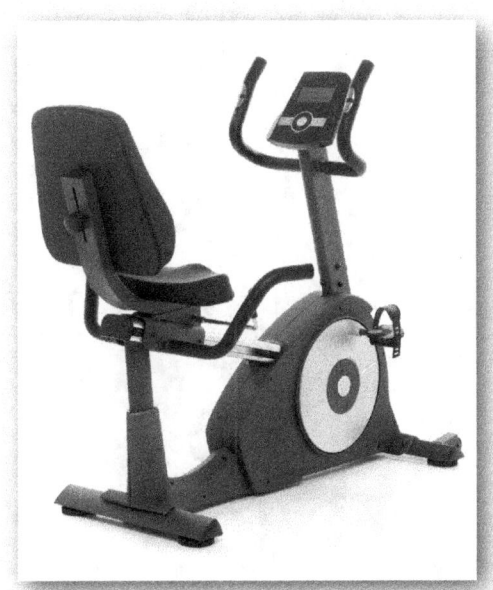

Upright bike

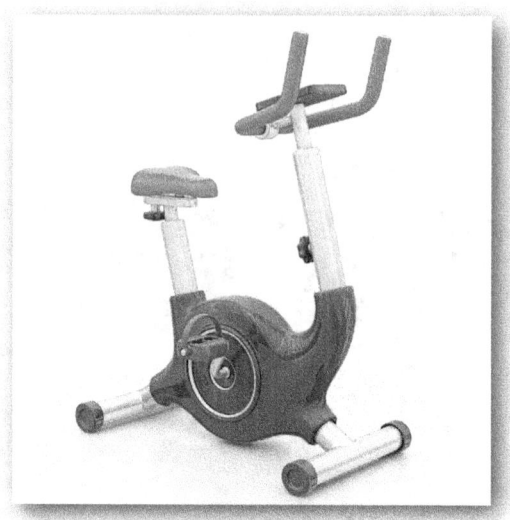

Stepper

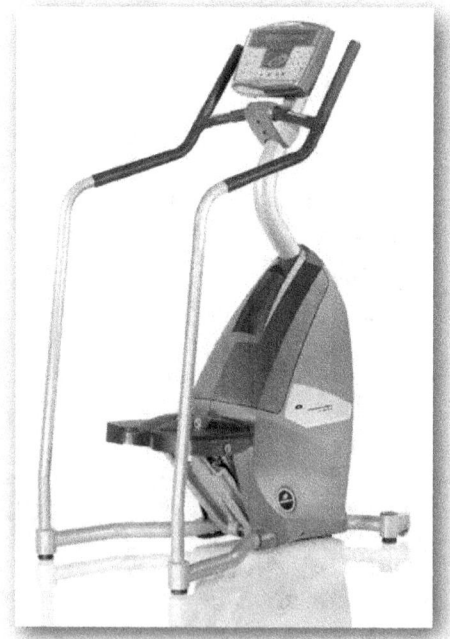

*Sunny health and fitness twister stepper with handle bar

Squats

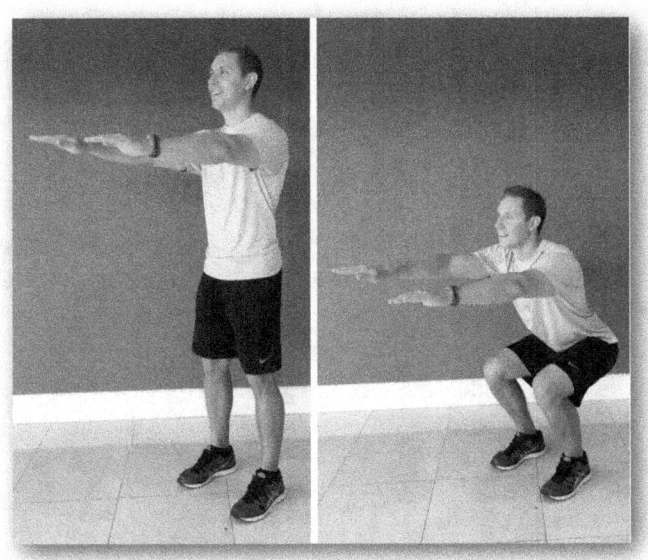

What muscle groups am I using when I do my cardio?

Heart, brain, quadriceps, hamstrings, gluteus maximus (butt), calves, core (abdominals, lower back, and obliques)

If I don't have access to a certain piece of cardio equipment, what should I use?

Treadmill = Walking/Jogging/Running
Elliptical = Cybex arc trainer
Cybex arc trainer = Elliptical
Recumbent bike = Upright bike
Upright bike = Recumbent bike
Jump-rope revolutions = Jumping jacks
Stepper = Squats

When should I stop working out?

- After you have completed everything on that day's workout
- If you injure yourself
- If you feel nauseous or dizzy

If you complete the workout in under thirty minutes, restart it from the beginning until your thirty-minute session is complete. When you feel that you need a rest, it is OK to take a 1-2 minute rest before resuming exercise. Pay attention to your body and listen to what it is telling you.

This book is evidence based and has flexibility. Consult your physician before exercising.

Cardio High

What is a cardio high?

After your body completes any fat-burning, high-intensity workout, you will feel an increase in energy levels, or what some call a "cardio high" or an "endorphin rush." Endorphins are produced in the brain, and these chemicals are sent throughout the body, which helps give relief from pain and can even help with the aging process. Endorphins produced by exercise can also enhance your immune system. Feel the rush: exercise not only benefits your body, but it benefits your mind as well. Exercise can help reduce anxiety, which, in turn, helps relieve stress and nervousness. This sensation can be triggered by other activities, including yoga, acupuncture, massage, and so forth.

"Exercise is a powerful drug. It seduces many with its zen-like state, a feeling that was coined the 'runner's high' in the 1970s. The lure of exercise can even turn enthusiasts into addicts." —Karen Asp

NEXT STEPS

What should I do when I finish all 365 workouts?
After you complete all 365 cardio workouts, I would recommend asking a friend or colleague to join you and repeat the workouts or mix them up in any order you desire. You have the flexibility to either complete the workouts in the same order or pick days at random and skip around. Remember that you can do cardio as minimally as two days per week and up to six days per week. Always take at least one day off per week to let your body rest and recover.

Get creative and have fun using this book!

Importance of Your Warm-Up

Your warm-up is important because it:

- Promotes blood flow through your body
- Increases your body temperature
- Loosens your muscles to prevent injury
- Reduces the likelihood of muscle soreness
- Enables you to perform better
- Prepares you mentally for your workout

Your warm-up consists of spending between 5-10 minutes on your favorite piece of cardio equipment. Pay attention to your warm-up target-heart-rate zone from the beginning of this book.

Your journey must begin from within. Let's go!

Day 1
____ *5-10 minute warm-up*
____ 1 mile on Cybex arc trainer
____ 9 minutes on treadmill, incline of "3"
____ 11 minutes on elliptical

Day 2
____ *5-10 minute warm-up*
____ 1 minute on treadmill (walk)
____ 1 minute on treadmill (jog/run)
____ Repeat for 8 minutes

____ 3 minutes on recumbent bike
____ 3 minutes on stepper
____ 33 push-ups (regular or modified)
____ Rest 1-2 minutes

____ 1 minute on treadmill (walk)
____ 1 minute on treadmill (jog/run)
____ Repeat for 16 minutes

"I really don't think I need buns of steel. I'd be happier with buns of cinnamon." — Ellen DeGeneres

DAY 3

____ *5-10 minute warm-up*
____ 2 miles on recumbent bike
____ 0.5 mile on Cybex arc trainer
____ 20 jumping jacks
____ 50 jump-rope revolutions
____ 2 minutes on stepper
____ 5 minutes on Cybex arc trainer
____ 20 jumping jacks
____ 20 push-ups (regular or modified)
____ 50 jump-rope revolutions
____ 2 minutes on treadmill (walk or jog)

DAY 4

____ *5-10 minute warm-up*
____ 9 minutes on recumbent bike
____ 8 minutes on upright bike
____ 7 minutes on elliptical
____ 6 minutes on recumbent bike
____ 5 minutes on elliptical

"Happiness is not in the mere possession of money; it lies in the joy of achievement, in the thrill of creative effort."—Franklin D. Roosevelt

DAY 5

____ *5-10 minute warm-up*
____ 2 minute jog/run on treadmill
____ 1 minute walk on treadmill
____ Repeat for 15 minutes

____ 7 minutes on stepper
____ 8 minutes on recumbent bike
____ 15 push-ups (regular or modified)

DAY 6

____ *5-10 minute warm-up*
____ 40 floors on stepper
____ 30 jump-rope revolutions
____ 20 floors on stepper
____ 1 mile on upright bike
____ 20 jump-rope revolutions
____ 30 floors on stepper
____ 40 jump-rope revolutions
____ 5 miles on upright bike
____ 40 push-ups (regular or modified)

"No one can make you feel inferior without your consent."—Eleanor Roosevelt

Day 7

____ *5-10 minute warm-up*
____ 7 minutes on treadmill
____ 7 minutes on upright bike
____ 7 minutes on recumbent bike
____ 7 minutes on treadmill, incline of "2"
____ 2 minutes on recumbent bike
____ 27 push-ups (regular or modified)

Day 8

____ *5-10 minute warm-up*
____ 3 minutes on recumbent bike
____ 5 floors on stepper
____ 10 push-ups (regular or modified)
____ 15 jumping jacks
____ 25 jump-rope revolutions
____ Rest 1-2 minutes

Repeat above grouping for 35 minutes

"There is only one way to happiness, and that is to cease worrying about things which are beyond the power of our will."—Epictetus

DAY 9

___ *5-10 minute warm-up*
___ 1 mile on recumbent bike
___ 1 mile on treadmill
___ 4 minutes on upright bike
___ 1 mile on elliptical
___ 1 mile on upright bike
___ 14 push-ups (regular or modified)

DAY 10

___ *5-10 minute warm-up*
___ 4 minutes on treadmill
___ 2 minutes on treadmill, incline of "6"
___ 2 minutes on treadmill
___ 2 minutes on treadmill, incline of "10"
___ 2 minutes on treadmill
___ 2 minutes on treadmill, incline of "4"
___ 2 minutes on treadmill
___ 2 minutes on treadmill, incline of "6"
___ 2 minutes on treadmill
___ 4 minutes on upright bike
___ 6 minutes on recumbent bike

"The purpose of life is life."—Karl Lagerfeld

DAY 11

_____ *5-10 minute warm-up*
_____ 1 mile on recumbent bike
_____ 50 floors on stepper
_____ 1 mile on upright bike
_____ 15 push-ups (regular or modified)
_____ 50 floors on stepper
_____ 1 mile on recumbent bike
_____ 50 floors on stepper
_____ 15 push-ups (regular or modified)

DAY 12

_____ *5-10 minute warm-up*
_____ 0.25 mile on treadmill
_____ 0.25 mile on elliptical
_____ 15 push-ups (regular or modified)
_____ Repeat for 25 minutes

_____ 25 squats
_____ 25 jumping jacks
_____ 25 floors on stepper
_____ 25 push-ups (regular or modified)

"Winners must have two things: definite goals and a burning desire to achieve them."—Brad Burden

Day 13

____ *5-10 minute warm-up*
____ 50 jump-rope revolutions
____ 10 floors on stepper
____ 40 jump-rope revolutions
____ 10 floors on stepper
____ 30 jump-rope revolutions
____ 10 floors on stepper
____ 20 jump-rope revolutions
____ 10 floors on stepper
____ 10 minutes on Cybex arc trainer
____ 50 push-ups (regular or modified)

Day 14

____ *5-10 minute warm-up*
____ 2 miles on treadmill
____ 5 minutes on recumbent bike
____ 5 minutes on treadmill (walk or jog)
____ 5 minutes on recumbent bike
____ 25 push-ups (regular or modified)

"Get out of the blocks, run your race, stay relaxed. If you run your race, you'll win. Channel your energy…Focus."—Carl Lewis

DAY 15

___ *5-10 minute warm-up*
___ 15 minutes on Cybex arc trainer
___ 7 floors on stepper
___ 10 minutes on Cybex arc trainer
___ 3 minutes on upright bike
___ 1 mile on recumbent bike
___ 15 push-ups (regular or modified)

DAY 16

___ *5-10 minute warm-up*
___ 2 minutes on treadmill
___ 4 minutes on treadmill, incline of "7"
___ 4 minutes on treadmill, incline of "5"
___ 4 minutes on treadmill, incline of "1"
___ Rest 1-2 minutes

___ 4 minutes on elliptical
___ 4 minutes on treadmill, incline of "5"
___ 4 minutes on treadmill, incline of "3"
___ 4 minutes on treadmill, incline of "1"
___ 2 minutes on treadmill (walk or jog)

"Change the fabric of your own soul and your own visions, and you change all."—Vachel Lindsay

DAY 17

____ *5-10 minute warm-up*
____ 20 jumping jacks
____ 20 jump-rope revolutions
____ 11 minutes on elliptical
____ Rest 1-2 minutes

____ 20 jumping jacks
____ 20 jump-rope revolutions
____ 11 minutes on elliptical
____ 20 push-ups (regular or modified)
____ Rest 1-2 minutes

____ 20 jumping jacks
____ 20 jump-rope revolutions
____ 11 minutes on elliptical

DAY 18

____ *5-10 minute warm-up*
____ 7 minutes on Cybex arc trainer
____ 4 miles on recumbent bike
____ 5 minutes on Cybex arc trainer
____ 2 miles on recumbent bike

"The greatest achievement of the human spirit is to live up to one's opportunities and make the most of one's resources."—Marquis de Vauvenargues

DAY 19

____ 5-10 minute warm-up
____ 10 floors on stepper
____ 3 minutes on treadmill
____ 20 floors on stepper
____ 3 minutes on treadmill
____ 30 floors on stepper
____ 3 minutes on treadmill
____ 40 floors on stepper
____ 3 minutes on treadmill
____ 50 push-ups (regular or modified)

DAY 20

____ 5-10 minute warm-up
____ Fun Workout!*

Aerobics 530	Backpacking 570	Badminton 370
Raking leaves 330	Dancing 450	Basketball 490
Boating 210	Boxing 735	Bowling 245
Canoeing 570	Fishing 250	Frisbee 250
Gardening 330	Golfing 370	Horseback riding 330
Ice skating 570	Mowing lawn 450	Racquetball 570
Soccer 570	Swimming laps 650	Tennis 570
Volleyball 430	Walking (moderate) 300	

Own activity: _____
Duration: _____

*Average calories burned in one hour by a 180-pound person are shown. (http://www.nutristrategy.com/activitylist4.htm)

"Where the old tracks are lost, new country is revealed with its wonders."
—Rabindranath Tagore

DAY 21

____ *5-10 minute warm-up*
____ 30 jumping jacks
____ 30 floors on stepper
____ 3 minutes on treadmill, incline of "3"
____ 3 miles on upright bike, level "3"
____ 30 jump-rope revolutions
____ 30 jumping jacks
____ 30 push-ups (regular or modified)

DAY 22

____ *5-10 minute warm-up*
____ 3 minutes on stepper
____ 6 minutes on treadmill
____ 60 jumping jacks
____ 4 minutes on stepper
____ 7 minutes on treadmill
____ 60 jumping jacks
____ 2 minutes on stepper
____ 8 minutes on treadmill

"Most people never run far enough on their first wind to find out they've got a second."—William James

DAY 23

____ *5-10 minute warm-up*
____ 13 minutes on treadmill, incline of "2"
____ 10 minutes on elliptical
____ 7 minutes on recumbent bike
____ 13 push-ups (regular or modified)

DAY 24

____ *5-10 minute warm-up*
____ 25 push-ups (regular or modified)
____ 100 floors on stepper (rest when needed)
____ 2 miles on upright bike
____ 5 minutes on treadmill
____ 25 floors on stepper

Remember to stay in your Target-Heart-Rate zone.

"The first thing is to love your sport. Never do it to please someone else. It has to be yours."—Peggy Fleming

DAY 25

___ *5-10 minute warm-up*
___ 1 minute on treadmill (walk)
___ 1 minute on treadmill (jog/run)
___ Repeat for 15 minutes

___ 6 minutes on recumbent bike
___ 1 mile on recumbent bike
___ 16 push-ups (regular or modified)
___ Rest 1-2 minutes

___ 1 minute on treadmill (walk)
___ 1 minute on treadmill (jog/run)
___ Repeat for 7 minutes

DAY 26

___ *5-10 minute warm-up*
___ 5 minutes on elliptical
___ 40 floors on stepper
___ 8 minutes on recumbent bike
___ 1 mile on treadmill
___ 10 jumping jacks

"Each day is a new life. Seize it. Live it."—David Guy Powers

DAY 27
____ *5-10 minute warm-up*
____ 20 jumping jacks
____ 4 minutes on treadmill
____ 20 jump-rope revolutions
____ 4 minutes on elliptical
____ 20 jumping jacks
____ 4 miles on upright bike
____ 20 jumping jacks
____ 4 minutes on elliptical
____ 20 push-ups (regular or modified)

DAY 28
____ *5-10 minute warm-up*
____ 3 miles on upright bike
____ 51 floors on stepper
____ 3 miles on upright bike
____ 51 jumping jacks
____ 3 miles on upright bike
____ 51 floors on stepper

"I attribute my success to this: I never gave or took any excuse."
—Florence Nightingale

Day 29

____ *5-10 minute warm-up*
____ 9 minutes on Cybex arc trainer
____ 10 floors on stepper
____ 5 minutes on treadmill
____ 20 jump-rope revolutions
____ 6 minutes on treadmill, incline of "3"
____ 3 minutes on upright bike
____ 5 jumping jacks
____ 2 minutes on treadmill

Day 30

____ *5-10 minute warm-up*
____ 14 minutes on Cybex arc trainer
____ 6 minutes on treadmill, incline of "5"
____ 2 minutes on stepper
____ 8 minutes on Cybex arc trainer
____ 14 push-ups (regular or modified)

"Just do your best today, and tomorrow will come...tomorrow's going to be a busy day, a happy day."—Helen Boehm

Day 31

____ *5-10 minute warm-up*
____ 10 floors on stepper
____ 10 minutes on elliptical
____ 10 floors on stepper
____ 10 minutes on elliptical
____ 10 floors on stepper
____ 10 minutes on elliptical
____ 10 floors on stepper

Day 32

____ *5-10 minute warm-up*
____ 4 minutes on treadmill, incline of "2"
____ 3 minutes on treadmill, incline of "4"
____ 2 minutes on treadmill, incline of "9"
____ 3 minutes on treadmill
____ Rest 1-2 minutes

____ 3 minutes on treadmill, incline of "6"
____ 2 minutes on treadmill, incline of "12"
____ 4 minutes on treadmill, incline of "2"
____ 3 minutes on treadmill, incline of "1"
____ 2 minutes on treadmill
____ Rest 1-2 minutes

____ 2 minutes on stepper
____ 8 minutes on recumbent bike
____ 28 push-ups (regular or modified)

"Knowledge of what is possible is the beginning of happiness."
—George Santayana

DAY 33

____ *5-10 minute warm-up*
____ 33 jump-rope revolutions
____ 4 minutes on upright bike
____ 2 minutes on upright bike, level "6"
____ 4 minutes on upright bike, level "8"
____ 2 minutes on upright bike, level "12"
____ 4 minutes on upright bike
____ 8 minutes on recumbent bike
____ 4 minutes on Cybex arc trainer

DAY 34

____ *5-10 minute warm-up*
____ 5 minutes on elliptical
____ 5 minutes on elliptical, level "8"
____ 5 minutes on treadmill
____ 25 push-ups (regular or modified)
____ 5 minutes on treadmill, incline of "8"
____ 5 minutes on stepper
____ 5 minutes on upright bike

"The way to develop self-confidence is to do the thing you fear and get a record of successful experiences behind you. Destiny is not a matter of chance, it is a matter of choice; it is not a thing to be waited for, it is a thing to be achieved."—William Jennings Bryan

Day 35

____ *5-10 minute warm-up*
____ 2 minutes on Cybex arc trainer
____ 10 minutes on recumbent bike
____ 10 push-ups (regular or modified)

____ 2 minutes on Cybex arc trainer
____ 10 minutes on recumbent bike
____ 2 minutes on Cybex arc trainer
____ 4 minutes on recumbent bike

Day 36

____ *5-10 minute warm-up*
____ 36 push-ups (regular or modified)
____ 9 minutes on treadmill
____ 9 minutes on elliptical
____ 9 minutes on upright bike
____ 3 minutes on treadmill
____ 36 push-ups (regular or modified)

"What you have to do and the way you have to do it is incredibly simple. Whether you are willing to do it is another matter."—Peter Drucker

DAY 37

___ *5-10 minute warm-up*
___ 25 minutes on stepper (take breaks when needed)
___ 5 minutes on recumbent bike
___ 25 jump-rope revolutions
___ 25 push-ups (regular or modified)

DAY 38

___ *5-10 minute warm-up*
___ 12 minutes on Cybex arc trainer
___ 10 minutes of jump rope (30 seconds on/30 seconds off)
___ 4 minutes on upright bike
___ 4 minutes on recumbent bike
___ 12 push-ups (regular or modified)

"Why not go out on a limb? That's where the fruit is."—Mark Twain

Day 39

___ 5-10 minute warm-up
___ 7 minutes on treadmill, incline of "4"
___ 36 floors on stepper
___ 1 mile on treadmill
___ 2 miles on upright bike
___ 36 push-ups (regular or modified)

Day 40

___ 5-10 minute warm-up
___ Fun Workout!*

Aerobics 530	Backpacking 570	Badminton 370
Raking leaves 330	Dancing 450	Basketball 490
Boating 210	Boxing 735	Bowling 245
Canoeing 570	Fishing 250	Frisbee 250
Gardening 330	Golfing 370	Horseback riding 330
Ice skating 570	Mowing lawn 450	Racquetball 570
Soccer 570	Swimming laps 650	Tennis 570
Volleyball 430	Walking (moderate) 300	

Own activity: _____
Duration: _____

*Average calories burned in one hour by a 180-pound person are shown. (http://www.nutristrategy.com/activitylist4.htm)

"Health is...a blessing that money cannot buy."—Izaak Walton

DAY 41

_____ *5-10 minute warm-up*
_____ 1 minute on treadmill, incline of "15"
_____ 3 minutes on treadmill, incline of "9"
_____ 3 minutes on treadmill, incline of "7"
_____ 3 minutes on treadmill, incline of "5"
_____ 5 minutes on upright bike, level "4"
_____ 5 minutes on upright bike, level "10"
_____ 5 minutes on upright bike, level "2"
_____ 5 minutes on upright bike

DAY 42

_____ *5-10 minute warm-up*
_____ 7 minutes on treadmill
_____ 7 minutes of push-ups (rest when needed)
_____ 7 minutes on elliptical
_____ 30 floors on stepper
_____ 60 jumping jacks
_____ 80 jump-rope revolutions
_____ 30 jumping jacks
_____ 30 push-ups (regular or modified)

"You must have discipline to have fun."—Julia Child

DAY 43

____ *5-10 minute warm-up*
____ 6 minutes on stepper
____ 6 push-ups (regular or modified)
____ 12 minutes on Cybex arc trainer
____ 12 minutes on recumbent bike
____ 6 minutes on stepper
____ 6 push-ups (regular or modified)

DAY 44

____ *5-10 minute warm-up*
____ 20 minutes on elliptical
____ 3 minutes on treadmill, incline of "12"
____ 3 minutes on treadmill, incline of "6"
____ 2 minutes on recumbent bike, level "12"
____ 2 miles on upright bike
____ 20 push-ups (regular or modified)

"Do each daily task the best we can; act as though the eyes of opportunity were always upon us."—William Feather

DAY 45
____ *5-10 minute warm-up*
____ Complete a 5K/10K race or (3.1/6.2 miles) on treadmill

Record your time: _____

DAY 46
____ *5-10 minute warm-up*
____ 50 jump-rope revolutions
____ 12 minutes on treadmill
____ 12 push-ups (regular or modified)
____ 25 jump-rope revolutions
____ 8 minutes on treadmill
____ 15 jump-rope revolutions
____ 6 minutes on treadmill
____ 10 jump-rope revolutions

"Knock the *t* off the 'can't.'"—George Reeves

DAY 47

____ *5-10 minute warm-up*
____ 3 minutes on recumbent bike
____ 6 minutes on elliptical
____ 3 minutes of push-ups (rest when needed)
____ 6 minutes on treadmill, incline of "6"
____ 12 minutes on elliptical
____ 36 push-ups (regular or modified)

DAY 48

____ *5-10 minute warm-up*
____ 6 minutes on upright bike
____ 3 minutes on upright bike, level "7"
____ 1 minute on upright bike, level "10"
____ 5 minutes on upright bike
____ 6 minutes on treadmill
____ 3 minutes on treadmill, incline of "3"
____ 1 minute on treadmill, incline of "12"
____ 5 minutes on treadmill

"Nothing great in the world has ever been accomplished without passion."—Georg Hegel

Day 49
____ *5-10 minute warm-up*
____ 44 jumping jacks
____ 11 minutes on Cybex arc trainer
____ 4 minutes on recumbent bike
____ 4 minutes Cybex arc trainer
____ 1 mile on elliptical
____ 1 minute of jump rope
____ 44 push-ups (regular or modified)

Day 50
____ *5-10 minute warm-up*
____ 7 floors on stepper
____ 2 minutes of jumping jacks
____ 4 minutes on treadmill, incline of "6"
____ 3 minutes on stepper
____ 1 minute on upright bike, level "13"
____ 2 minutes of jumping jacks
____ 7 floors on stepper
____ 8 minutes on treadmill
____ 7 minutes on upright bike
____ 1 minute on treadmill, incline of "15"

"Sleep is that golden chain that ties health and our bodies together."
—Thomas Dekker

DAY 51

____ *5-10 minute warm-up*
____ 2 minutes on elliptical
____ 9 minutes on upright bike
____ 10 minutes on Cybex arc trainer
____ 4 minutes on elliptical
____ 5 minutes on treadmill, incline of "3"
____ 10 push-ups (regular or modified)

DAY 52

____ *5-10 minute warm-up*
____ 7 floors on stepper
____ 2 minutes on Cybex arc trainer
____ 4 minutes on recumbent bike
____ 7 minutes on treadmill
____ 2 minutes on Cybex arc trainer
____ 8 floors on stepper
____ 4 minutes on treadmill, incline of "4"
____ 2 minutes of jumping jacks
____ 6 floors on stepper
____ 4 minutes on treadmill

"If you want to stand out, don't be different, be outstanding."
—Meredith West

DAY 53

____ *5-10 minute warm-up*
____ 1 minute on treadmill (walk)
____ 1 minute on treadmill (jog/run)
____ Repeat for 16 minutes

____ 1 mile on recumbent bike
____ 4 minutes on upright bike
____ Rest 1-2 minutes

____ 1 minute on treadmill (walk)
____ 1 minute on treadmill (jog/run)
____ Repeat for 7 minutes

DAY 54

____ *5-10 minute warm-up*
____ 1 minute of jumping jacks
____ 1 minute of jump rope
____ 5 minutes on recumbent bike
____ 15 push-ups (regular or modified)

____ Repeat above grouping for 30 minutes

"The key to change...is to let go of fear."—Rosanne Cash

DAY 55

____ *5-10 minute warm-up*
____ 1 mile on treadmill
____ 4 minutes on recumbent bike
____ 5 minutes on elliptical
____ 9 minutes on recumbent bike
____ 4 minutes on treadmill, incline of "4"

DAY 56

____ *5-10 minute warm-up*
____ 20 jump-rope revolutions
____ 8 minutes on treadmill
____ 20 jump-rope revolutions
____ 8 minutes on treadmill
____ 20 jump-rope revolutions
____ 8 minutes on treadmill
____ 20 jump-rope revolutions
____ 8 push-ups (regular or modified)
____ 20 jump-rope revolutions

"It's quite possible to leave your home for a walk in the early morning air and return a different person—beguiled, enchanted."—Mary Chase

DAY 57
____ *5-10 minute warm-up*
____ 10 minutes on Cybex arc trainer
____ 25 floors on stepper
____ 6 minutes on Cybex arc trainer
____ 25 floors on stepper
____ 4 minutes on Cybex arc trainer
____ 25 floors on stepper
____ 10 push-ups (regular or modified)

DAY 58
____ *5-10 minute warm-up*
____ 4 minutes on treadmill
____ 2 minutes on treadmill, incline of "2"
____ 1 minute on treadmill
____ 4 minutes on treadmill, incline of "4"
____ 2 minutes on treadmill
____ 6 minutes on treadmill, incline of "6"
____ 1 minute on treadmill
____ 8 minutes on treadmill, incline of "8"
____ 2 minutes on treadmill

"I want to do it because I want to do it."—Amelia Earhart

DAY 59

___ *5-10 minute warm-up*
___ 3 minutes on stepper
___ 1 mile on recumbent bike
___ 2 minutes on stepper
___ 4 minutes on recumbent bike
___ 1 minute on stepper
___ 1 mile on recumbent bike
___ 9 minutes on elliptical

DAY 60

___ *5-10 minute warm-up*
___ Fun Workout!*

Aerobics 530	Backpacking 570	Badminton 370
Raking leaves 330	Dancing 450	Basketball 490
Boating 210	Boxing 735	Bowling 245
Canoeing 570	Fishing 250	Frisbee 250
Gardening 330	Golfing 370	Horseback riding 330
Ice skating 570	Mowing lawn 450	Racquetball 570
Soccer 570	Swimming laps 650	Tennis 570
Volleyball 430	Walking (moderate) 300	

Own activity: _____

Duration: _____

*Average calories burned in one hour by a 180-pound person are shown. (http://www.nutristrategy.com/activitylist4.htm)

"To grow and know what one is growing towards—that is the source of all strength and confidence in life."—James Baillie

DAY 61

____ *5-10 minute warm-up*
____ 8 minutes on recumbent bike
____ 80 jump-rope revolutions
____ 8 minutes on treadmill, incline of "5"
____ 80 jump-rope revolutions
____ 8 minutes on treadmill, incline of "3"
____ 80 jump-rope revolutions

DAY 62

____ *5-10 minute warm-up*
____ 14 minutes on elliptical
____ 38 jumping jacks
____ 14 minutes on recumbent bike
____ 38 jumping jacks
____ 14 push-ups (regular or modified)
____ 38 jumping jacks

"The chief function of the body is to carry the brain around."—Thomas Edison

DAY 63

____ *5-10 minute warm-up*
____ 7 minutes on Cybex arc trainer
____ 3 minutes on treadmill, incline of "6"
____ 44 floors on stepper
____ 6 minutes on treadmill
____ 7 minutes on elliptical
____ 2 minutes on upright bike

DAY 64

____ *5-10 minute warm-up*
____ 20 minutes on elliptical
____ 5 minutes on treadmill, incline of "5"
____ 5 minutes on treadmill, incline of "2"
____ 20 push-ups (regular or modified)

"Ability is what you're capable of doing. Motivation determines what you do. Attitude determines how well you do it."—Lou Holtz

DAY 65

____ *5-10 minute warm-up*

____ 1 mile on recumbent bike

____ 1 mile on upright bike

____ 1 mile on treadmill (walk/jog)

____ 1 mile on upright bike

____ 1 mile on recumbent bike

____ 5 minutes on treadmill, incline of "5"

DAY 66

____ *5-10 minute warm-up*

____ 7 minutes on Cybex arc trainer

____ 7 minutes on treadmill

____ 5 minutes on Cybex arc trainer

____ 5 minutes on treadmill, incline of "5"

____ 3 minutes on Cybex arc trainer

____ 3 minutes on treadmill

"Even if you're on the right track, you'll get run over if you just sit there."—Will Rogers

DAY 67

____ *5-10 minute warm-up*
____ 2 miles on recumbent bike
____ 4 minutes on elliptical
____ 2 miles on upright bike
____ 4 minutes on elliptical
____ 2 miles on recumbent bike
____ 24 push-ups (regular or modified)

DAY 68

____ *5-10 minute warm-up*
____ 3 minutes on recumbent bike
____ 1 minute of jumping jacks
____ 2 minutes of jump rope (rest when needed)
____ 5 minutes on elliptical
____ 3 minutes on treadmill, incline of "3"
____ 8 minutes on recumbent bike
____ 3 minutes on upright bike

"Our dilemma is that we hate change and love it at the same time; what we really want is for things to remain the same but get better."
—Sydney J. Harris

DAY 69

___ *5-10 minute warm-up*
___ 8 minutes on upright bike
___ 8 minutes on treadmill
___ 8 minutes on Cybex arc trainer
___ 58 jump-rope revolutions
___ 89 jumping jacks

DAY 70

___ *5-10 minute warm-up*
___ 3 minutes on elliptical
___ 2 minutes on stepper
___ 1 mile on upright bike

___ Repeat above grouping 5 times

"Nothing is impossible; the word itself says 'I'm possible'!"—Audrey Hepburn

DAY 71

___ *5-10 minute warm-up*
___ 10 minutes on Cybex arc trainer
___ 4 minutes on recumbent bike
___ 8 minutes on treadmill
___ 4 minutes on Cybex arc trainer
___ 4 minutes on treadmill, incline of "8"
___ 10 push-ups (regular or modified)

DAY 72

___ *5-10 minute warm-up*
___ 7 minutes on treadmill, incline of "2"
___ 7 minutes on elliptical
___ 70 jumping jacks
___ Rest 1-2 minutes

___ 80 jumping jacks
___ 3 miles on upright bike
___ 33 push-ups (regular or modified)

"I never dreamed about success, I worked for it."—Estee Lauder

DAY 73

___ *5-10 minute warm-up*
___ 17 minutes on treadmill
___ 8 minutes on recumbent bike
___ 33 floors on stepper
___ 17 push-ups (regular or modified)

DAY 74

___ *5-10 minute warm-up*
___ 3 minutes on Cybex arc trainer
___ 4 minutes on upright bike
___ 2 minutes on stepper
___ 2 minutes on treadmill, incline of "10"
___ 1 mile on upright bike
___ 7 minutes on Cybex arc trainer
___ 7 minutes on elliptical

"I don't exercise. If God wanted me to bend over, he would have put diamonds on the floor."—Joan Rivers

DAY 75

____ *5-10 minute warm-up*
____ 1 minute on treadmill (walk)
____ 1 minute on treadmill (jog/run)
____ Repeat for 11 minutes

____ 2 miles on recumbent bike
____ Rest 1-2 minutes

____ 1 minute on treadmill (walk)
____ 1 minute on treadmill (jog/run)
____ Repeat for 12 minutes

DAY 76

____ *5-10 minute warm-up*
____ 5 minutes on Cybex arc trainer
____ 20 jumping jacks
____ 9 minutes on elliptical
____ 1 mile on recumbent bike
____ 7 minutes on Cybex arc trainer
____ 4 minutes on stepper

"The secret of change is to focus all your energy not on fighting the old, but on building the new."—Dan Millman

DAY 77

___ *5-10 minute warm-up*
___ 2 minutes on recumbent bike
___ 5 miles on upright bike
___ 40 floors on stepper
___ 84 jump-rope revolutions
___ 2 minutes on recumbent bike

DAY 78

___ *5-10 minute warm-up*
___ 75 jump-rope revolutions
___ 3 minutes on Cybex arc trainer
___ 75 jump-rope revolutions
___ 4 minutes on Cybex arc trainer
___ 50 jump-rope revolutions
___ 5 minutes on Cybex arc trainer
___ 50 jump-rope revolutions
___ 4 minutes on Cybex arc trainer
___ 25 jump-rope revolutions
___ 3 minutes on Cybex arc trainer
___ 25 jump-rope revolutions

"Love yourself enough to live a healthy lifestyle."—Anonymous

DAY 79

____ *5-10 minute warm-up*
____ 10 minutes on elliptical
____ 10 minutes on treadmill
____ 10 minutes on upright bike
____ 100 floors on the stepper (rest when needed)
____ 1 minute on treadmill

DAY 80

____ *5-10 minute warm-up*
____ Fun Workout!*

Aerobics 530	Backpacking 570	Badminton 370
Raking leaves 330	Dancing 450	Basketball 490
Boating 210	Boxing 735	Bowling 245
Canoeing 570	Fishing 250	Frisbee 250
Gardening 330	Golfing 370	Horseback riding 330
Ice skating 570	Mowing lawn 450	Racquetball 570
Soccer 570	Swimming laps 650	Tennis 570
Volleyball 430	Walking (moderate) 300	

Own activity: _____
Duration: _____

*Average calories burned in one hour by a 180-pound person are shown. (http://www.nutristrategy.com/activitylist4.htm)

"Enjoy your own life without comparing it with that of another."
—Marquis de Condorcet

DAY 81

____ *5-10 minute warm-up*
____ 70 jump-rope revolutions
____ 7 minutes on elliptical
____ 60 jump-rope revolutions
____ 6 minutes on elliptical
____ 50 jump-rope revolutions
____ 5 minutes on elliptical
____ 40 jump-rope revolutions
____ 4 minutes on elliptical
____ 30 jump-rope revolutions
____ 3 minutes on elliptical
____ 20 jump-rope revolutions
____ 2 minutes on elliptical
____ 2 minutes on recumbent bike

DAY 82

____ *5-10 minute warm-up*
____ 1 mile on upright bike
____ 70 jumping jacks
____ 33 floors on stepper
____ 1 mile on treadmill
____ 1 mile on upright bike
____ 33 push-ups (regular or modified)
____ 70 jumping jacks

"Sometimes your joy is the source of your smile, but sometimes your smile can be the source of your joy."—Thich Nhat Hanh

Day 83
___ *5-10 minute warm-up*
___ 3 minutes on stepper
___ 2 minutes on recumbent bike
___ 1 mile on Cybex arc trainer
___ 8 minutes on treadmill
___ 8 minutes on Cybex arc trainer
___ 80 jump-rope revolutions

Day 84
___ *5-10 minute warm-up*
___ 20 minutes on treadmill
___ 4 minutes on recumbent bike
___ 4 minutes on treadmill, incline of "4"
___ 2 minutes on recumbent bike
___ 20 push-ups (regular or modified)

"First say to yourself what you would be, and then do what you have to do."—Epictetus

DAY 85

____ *5-10 minute warm-up*
____ 1 mile on elliptical
____ 9 minutes on stepper
____ 8 minutes on upright bike
____ 4 minutes on elliptical

DAY 86

____ *5-10 minute warm-up*
____ 0.5 mile on treadmill
____ 0.5 mile on Cybex arc trainer
____ 0.25 mile on treadmill
____ 0.25 mile on Cybex arc trainer
____ 125 jump-rope revolutions
____ 125 jumping jacks

"When you want to succeed as bad as you want to breathe, then you'll be successful." —Eric Thomas

DAY 87
____ *5-10 minute warm-up*
____ 3 miles on recumbent bike
____ 3 miles on upright bike
____ 2 miles on recumbent bike
____ 2 miles on upright bike
____ 1 mile on recumbent bike
____ 1 mile on upright bike

DAY 88
____ *5-10 minute warm-up*
____ 25 jumping jacks
____ 50 jump-rope revolutions
____ 15 floors on stepper
____ Repeat 5 times

"I have found that if you love life, life will love you back."—Arthur Rubinstein

DAY 89

___ *5-10 minute warm-up*

___ 6 minutes on treadmill, incline of "2"

___ 2 minutes on treadmill, incline of "6"

___ 7 minutes on treadmill, incline of "3"

___ 3 minutes on treadmill, incline of "7"

___ 3 miles on upright bike

DAY 90

___ *5-10 minute warm-up*

___ Complete a 5K/10K race or (3.1/6.2 miles) on treadmill

Record your time: _____

"The difference between ordinary and extraordinary is that little extra."—Jimmy Johnson

DAY 91

___ *5-10 minute warm-up*
___ 9 minutes on treadmill
___ 45 seconds of jumping jacks
___ 2 minutes on treadmill, incline of "4.5"
___ 45 seconds of jumping jacks
___ 2 minutes on treadmill, incline of "7.5"
___ 45 seconds of jumping jacks
___ 3 minutes on treadmill, incline of "2.5"
___ 45 seconds of jumping jacks
___ 0.5 mile on elliptical
___ 1 mile on recumbent bike

DAY 92

___ *5-10 minute warm-up*
___ 5 minutes on stepper
___ 7 minutes on upright bike
___ 12 minutes on Cybex arc trainer
___ 5 minutes on stepper
___ 7 minutes on upright bike

"Give every day the chance to become the most beautiful day of your life."—Mark Twain

Day 93

___ *5-10 minute warm-up*
___ 2 miles on recumbent bike
___ 1 mile on treadmill
___ 4 minutes on Cybex arc trainer
___ 9 minutes on treadmill, incline of "4"
___ 1 mile on recumbent bike

Day 94

___ *5-10 minute warm-up*
___ 1 minute walk on treadmill
___ 1 minute jog/run on treadmill
___ Repeat for 18 minutes

___ Rest 1-2 minutes
___ 1 mile on upright bike
___ 8 minutes on stepper (rest when needed)
___ 18 push-ups (regular or modified)

"Concentrate on finding your goal, then concentrate on reaching it."
—Colonel Michael Friedsam

DAY 95
____ *5-10 minute warm-up*
____ 4 minutes on elliptical
____ 7 minutes on Cybex arc trainer
____ 2 miles on elliptical
____ 90 jumping jacks

DAY 96
____ *5-10 minute warm-up*
____ 5 minutes on treadmill, incline of "3"
____ 6 minutes on recumbent bike
____ 2 minutes on Cybex arc trainer
____ 9 minutes on treadmill
____ 1 mile on Cybex arc trainer
____ 10 jump-rope revolutions

"Accurate information is a key part of motivation."—Mary Ann Allison

Day 97

____ *5-10 minute warm-up*
____ 4 minutes on treadmill
____ 5 minutes on elliptical
____ 4 minutes on treadmill, incline of "4"
____ 5 minutes on elliptical, level "6"
____ 4 minutes on treadmill, incline of "8"
____ 5 minutes on elliptical, level "10"
____ 6 minutes on upright bike, level "6"

Day 98

____ *5-10 minute warm-up*
____ 30 jumping jacks
____ 6 minutes on recumbent bike
____ 8 minutes on upright bike
____ 30 jumping jacks
____ 4 minutes on recumbent bike
____ 6 minutes on upright bike
____ 30 jumping jacks
____ 2 minutes on recumbent bike
____ 4 minutes on upright bike
____ 30 jumping jacks

"Decisions determine destiny."—Frederick Speakman

DAY 99

____ *5-10 minute warm-up*
____ 10 minutes on Cybex arc trainer
____ 5 minutes on treadmill
____ 10 push-ups (regular or modified)
____ 5 minutes on Cybex arc trainer
____ 10 minutes on treadmill

DAY 100

____ *5-10 minute warm-up*
____ 100 jumping jacks
____ 100 floors on stepper (rest when needed)
____ 100 jump-rope revolutions
____ 10 minutes on treadmill

"Be yourself; everyone else is already taken."—Oscar Wilde

DAY 101
____ 5-10 minute warm-up
____ Fun Workout!*

Aerobics 530	Backpacking 570	Badminton 370
Raking leaves 330	Dancing 450	Basketball 490
Boating 210	Boxing 735	Bowling 245
Canoeing 570	Fishing 250	Frisbee 250
Gardening 330	Golfing 370	Horseback riding 330
Ice skating 570	Mowing lawn 450	Racquetball 570
Soccer 570	Swimming laps 650	Tennis 570
Volleyball 430	Walking (moderate) 300	

Own activity: _____
Duration: _____

*Average calories burned in one hour by a 180-pound person are shown. (http://www.nutristrategy.com/activitylist4.htm)

DAY 102
____ 5-10 minute warm-up
____ 1 minute on treadmill (walk)
____ 1 minute on treadmill (jog/run)
____ Repeat for 8 minutes

____ 10 minutes on recumbent bike
____ 1 mile on upright bike
____ 10 push-ups (regular or modified)

____ 1 minute on treadmill (walk)
____ 1 minute on treadmill (jog/run)
____ Repeat for 9 minutes

"There is no substitute for hard work."—Thomas Edison

DAY 103

___ *5-10 minute warm-up*
___ 6 minutes on elliptical
___ 60 jump-rope revolutions
___ 4 minutes on elliptical
___ 40 jump-rope revolutions
___ 3 minutes on elliptical
___ 30 jump-rope revolutions
___ 2 minutes on stepper
___ 2 minutes on elliptical, level "10"
___ 8 minutes on treadmill

DAY 104

___ *5-10 minute warm-up*
___ 0.5 mile on recumbent bike
___ 0.5 mile on Cybex arc trainer
___ 0.5 mile on treadmill
___ 25 jumping jacks
___ 1 mile on upright bike
___ 1 mile on recumbent bike
___ 1 mile on Cybex arc trainer
___ 0.5 mile on treadmill
___ 25 jumping jacks
___ 1 mile on upright bike

"Unless you give yourself to some great cause, you haven't even begun to live." —William P. Merrill

DAY 105

____ *5-10 minute warm-up*
____ 5 minutes on treadmill
____ 1 minute on treadmill, incline of "10"
____ 4 minutes on treadmill
____ 1 minute on treadmill, incline of "9"
____ 5 minutes on treadmill
____ 1 minute on treadmill, incline of "8"
____ 4 minutes on treadmill
____ 1 minute on treadmill, incline of "7"
____ 6 miles on recumbent bike

DAY 106

____ *5-10 minute warm-up*
____ 40 floors on stepper
____ 40 jumping jacks
____ 3 miles on recumbent bike
____ 1 mile on elliptical
____ 15 floors on stepper
____ 15 jumping jacks
____ 1 mile on elliptical

"Optimism is an intellectual choice."—Diana Schneider

DAY 107

____ *5-10 minute warm-up*
____ 7 minutes on treadmill
____ 7 minutes on upright bike
____ 7 minutes on recumbent bike
____ 3 minutes on treadmill, incline of "6"
____ 17 jump-rope revolutions
____ 6 minutes on upright bike
____ 107 jump-rope revolutions
____ 17 push-ups (regular or modified)

DAY 108

____ *5-10 minute warm-up*
____ 8 minutes on treadmill, incline of "2"
____ 5 minutes on Cybex arc trainer
____ 1 minute of jump rope
____ Rest 1-2 minutes

____ 0.8 mile on treadmill
____ 0.5 mile on Cybex arc trainer
____ 1 minute of jump rope

"People often say that motivation doesn't last. Well, neither does bathing – that's why we recommend it daily." —Zig Ziglar

DAY 109

____ *5-10 minute warm-up*
____ 4 minutes on elliptical
____ 4 minutes on stepper
____ 4 minutes on elliptical
____ 4 minutes on stepper
____ 2 minutes on recumbent bike
____ 2 minutes of jump rope
____ 2 minutes on recumbent bike
____ 2 minutes of jump rope
____ 2 minutes on recumbent bike
____ 2 minutes of jump rope
____ 2 minutes on upright bike

DAY 110

____ *5-10 minute warm-up*
____ 7 jumping jacks
____ 7 minutes on upright bike
____ 7 minutes on treadmill
____ 7 minutes on recumbent bike
____ 9 jumping jacks
____ 1 mile on upright bike
____ 1 mile on recumbent bike

"For many men, the acquisition of wealth does not end their troubles, it only changes them."—Seneca

DAY 111

___ *5-10 minute warm-up*
___ 8 minutes on treadmill
___ 4 miles on upright bike
___ 32 jump-rope revolutions
___ 4 minutes on treadmill, incline of "4"

DAY 112

___ *5-10 minute warm-up*
___ 15 floors on stepper
___ 0.5 mile on elliptical
___ 15 floors on stepper
___ 0.5 mile on elliptical
___ 30 floors on stepper
___ 0.3 mile on treadmill, incline of "3"
___ 3 minutes on stepper
___ 9 minutes on treadmill

"Lack of activity destroys the good condition of every human being, while movement and methodical physical exercise save it and preserve it."—Plato

DAY 113
____ *5-10 minute warm-up*
____ 25 push-ups (regular or modified)
____ 1 mile on elliptical
____ 1 mile on recumbent bike
____ 1 mile on elliptical
____ 1 mile on Cybex arc trainer
____ 25 floors on stepper
____ 25 push-ups (regular or modified)

DAY 114
____ *5-10 minute warm-up*
____ 10 minutes on treadmill
____ 45 jumping jacks
____ 8 minutes on upright bike
____ 35 jumping jacks
____ 6 minutes on treadmill
____ 25 jump-rope revolutions
____ 4 minutes on upright bike
____ 15 jump-rope revolutions

"Food is the most widely abused anti-anxiety drug in America, and exercise is the most potent, yet underutilized antidepressant."—Bill Phillips

DAY 115

____ *5-10 minute warm-up*
____ 3 minutes on treadmill
____ 4 minutes on elliptical
____ 2 minutes on elliptical, level "10"
____ 4 minutes on elliptical
____ 2 minutes on elliptical, level "13"
____ 4 minutes on elliptical
____ 2 minutes on elliptical, level "7"
____ 4 minutes on elliptical
____ 5 minutes on treadmill

DAY 116

____ *5-10 minute warm-up*
____ 4 minutes on Cybex arc trainer
____ 10 minutes on treadmill
____ 100 jump-rope revolutions
____ 10 minutes on stepper (rest when needed)

"Energy and persistence conquer all things."—Benjamin Franklin

DAY 117
____ *5-10 minute warm-up*
____ 8 minutes on recumbent bike
____ 16 jumping jacks
____ 1 mile on upright bike
____ 9 minutes on elliptical
____ 8 minutes on treadmill
____ 3 minutes of jump rope

DAY 118
____ *5-10 minute warm-up*
____ 6 minutes on elliptical
____ 2 miles on treadmill
____ 20 jump-rope revolutions
____ 20 push-ups (regular or modified)

"Plenty of people miss their share of happiness, not because they never found it, but because they didn't stop to enjoy it."—William Feather

DAY 119

____ *5-10 minute warm-up*
____ 2 minutes on Cybex arc trainer
____ 11 minutes on upright bike
____ 20 floors on stepper
____ 10 minutes on Cybex arc trainer

DAY 120

____ *5-10 minute warm-up*
____ Fun Workout!*

Aerobics 530	Backpacking 570	Badminton 370
Raking leaves 330	Dancing 450	Basketball 490
Boating 210	Boxing 735	Bowling 245
Canoeing 570	Fishing 250	Frisbee 250
Gardening 330	Golfing 370	Horseback riding 330
Ice skating 570	Mowing lawn 450	Racquetball 570
Soccer 570	Swimming laps 650	Tennis 570
Volleyball 430	Walking (moderate) 300	

Own activity: _____
Duration: _____

*Average calories burned in one hour by a 180-pound person are shown. (http://www.nutristrategy.com/activitylist4.htm)

"Learn to let go. That is the key to happiness."—Buddha

DAY 121

____ *5-10 minute warm-up*
____ 95 jumping jacks
____ 8 minutes on elliptical
____ 8 minutes on recumbent bike
____ 75 jumping jacks
____ 4 minutes on recumbent bike
____ 4 minutes on elliptical
____ 55 jumping jacks

DAY 122

____ *5-10 minute warm-up*
____ 11 minutes on Cybex arc trainer
____ 21 floors on stepper
____ 1 mile on upright bike
____ 9 minutes on treadmill
____ 8 minutes on Cybex arc trainer
____ 4 minutes on stepper

"Pride…is the direct appreciation of oneself."—Arthur Schopenhauer

DAY 123

____ *5-10 minute warm-up*
____ 7 jumping jacks
____ 2 minutes on elliptical
____ 4 minutes on recumbent bike
____ 7 minutes on treadmill, incline of "2"
____ 7 minutes on recumbent bike, level "4"
____ 7 minutes on treadmill
____ 7 minutes on elliptical
____ 8 jumping jacks
____ 1 minute on elliptical

DAY 124

____ *5-10 minute warm-up*
____ 50 jump-rope revolutions
____ 1 mile on Cybex arc trainer
____ 50 jump-rope revolutions
____ 1 mile on elliptical
____ 50 jump-rope revolutions
____ 1 mile on Cybex arc trainer
____ 50 jump-rope revolutions

"Pain is no longer pain when it is past."—Margaret Junkin Preston

DAY 125

____ *5-10 minute warm-up*
____ 1 minute on treadmill (walk)
____ 1 minute on treadmill (jog/run)
____ Repeat for 8 minutes

____ Rest 1-2 minutes
____ 1 mile on recumbent bike
____ 7 minutes on upright bike

____ 1 minute on treadmill (walk)
____ 1 minute on treadmill (jog/run)
____ Repeat for 12 minutes

DAY 126

____ *5-10 minute warm-up*
____ 0.5 mile on treadmill
____ 1 mile on recumbent bike
____ 0.5 mile on treadmill, incline of "4"
____ 1 mile on recumbent bike
____ Rest 1-2 minutes

____ 25 jumping jacks
____ 25 jump-rope revolutions
____ 25 jumping jacks
____ 25 jump-rope revolutions
____ Rest 1-2 minutes

____ 0.5 mile on treadmill
____ 1 mile on recumbent bike
____ 0.5 mile on treadmill, incline of "4"
____ 1 mile on recumbent bike

"Do one thing every day that scares you."—Eleanor Roosevelt

DAY 127

____ *5-10 minute warm-up*
____ 7 minutes on Cybex arc trainer
____ 3 minutes on upright bike
____ 3 miles on recumbent bike
____ 3 minutes on Cybex arc trainer
____ 3 minutes on upright bike
____ 7 minutes on treadmill

DAY 128

____ *5-10 minute warm-up*
____ 88 jumping jacks
____ 77 jump-rope revolutions
____ 66 jumping jacks
____ 55 jump-rope revolutions
____ 44 jumping jacks
____ 33 floors on stepper
____ 22 jump-rope revolutions
____ 11 jumping jacks
____ 1 mile on treadmill

"Experience tells you what to do; confidence allows you to do it."—
Stan Smith

DAY 129
____ *5-10 minute warm-up*
____ 16 minutes on elliptical
____ 7 minutes on treadmill
____ 7 minutes on recumbent bike

DAY 130
____ *5-10 minute warm-up*
____ 13 floors on stepper
____ 3 minutes on treadmill, incline of "13"
____ 3 minutes on treadmill
____ Rest 1-2 minutes

____ 13 floors on stepper
____ 3 minutes on treadmill, incline of "13"
____ 3 minutes on treadmill
____ Rest 1-2 minutes

____ 1 mile on upright bike
____ 3 minutes on recumbent bike, level "13"
____ 1 mile on upright bike
____ 3 minutes on recumbent bike, level "13"

"In the long run we shape our lives, and we shape ourselves. The process never ends until we die. And the choices we make are ultimately our own responsibility."—Eleanor Roosevelt

Day 131
____ *5-10 minute warm-up*
____ 9 minutes on Cybex arc trainer
____ 7 minutes on elliptical
____ 5 minutes on stepper
____ 3 minutes on Cybex arc trainer
____ 1 mile on recumbent bike

Day 132
____ *5-10 minute warm-up*
____ 25 jump-rope revolutions
____ 5 minutes on treadmill, incline of "5"
____ 25 jump-rope revolutions
____ 4 minutes on treadmill, incline of "4"
____ 50 jump-rope revolutions
____ 3 minutes on treadmill, incline of "3"
____ 50 jump-rope revolutions
____ 2 minutes on treadmill, incline of "2"
____ 50 jump-rope revolutions
____ 1 minute on treadmill, incline of "1"
____ 100 jump-rope revolutions
____ 5 minutes on treadmill

"What great thing would you attempt if you knew you could not fail?"—Robert Schuller

DAY 133

____ *5-10 minute warm-up*
____ 4 minutes on treadmill, incline of "7"
____ 4 minutes on Cybex arc trainer
____ 4 minutes on elliptical
____ 4 minutes on treadmill, incline of "4"
____ 4 minutes on Cybex arc trainer
____ 1 mile on treadmill, incline of "4"

DAY 134

____ *5-10 minute warm-up*
____ 10 jumping jacks
____ 3 minutes on recumbent bike, level "16"
____ 20 jumping jacks
____ 3 minutes on recumbent bike, level "14"
____ 30 jumping jacks
____ 3 minutes on recumbent bike, level "12"
____ 40 jumping jacks
____ 4 minutes on recumbent bike, level "10"
____ 50 jumping jacks
____ 4 minutes on recumbent bike, level "8"
____ 60 jumping jacks
____ 4 minutes on recumbent bike, level "6"
____ 70 jumping jacks
____ 5 minutes on recumbent bike, level "4"
____ 80 jumping jacks
____ 5 minutes on recumbent bike, level "2"
____ 90 jumping jacks
____ 5 minutes on recumbent bike
____ 100 jumping jacks

"Without discipline, there's no life at all."—Katharine Hepburn

DAY 135

___ *5-10 minute warm-up*
___ Complete a 5K/10K race or (3.1/6.2 miles) on treadmill

Record your time: _____

DAY 136

___ *5-10 minute warm-up*
___ 5 minutes on recumbent bike
___ 6 minutes on elliptical
___ 2 miles on upright bike
___ 9 minutes on recumbent bike
___ 110 jump-rope revolutions

"What a man accomplishes in a day depends upon the way in which he approaches his tasks. When we accept tough jobs as a challenge to our ability and wade into them with joy and enthusiasm, miracles can happen."—Arland Gilbert

DAY 137

____ *5-10 minute warm-up*
____ 8 minutes on elliptical
____ 4 minutes on upright bike
____ 32 floors on stepper
____ 80 jump-rope revolutions
____ 80 jumping jacks
____ 4 minutes on upright bike
____ 8 minutes on elliptical

DAY 138

____ *5-10 minute warm-up*
____ 4 miles on recumbent bike
____ 1 mile on Cybex arc trainer
____ 1 mile on recumbent bike
____ 4 minutes on upright bike

"We cannot do everything at once, but we can do something at once."—Calvin Coolidge

DAY 139

____ *5-10 minute warm-up*
____ 24 floors on stepper
____ 2.4 miles on treadmill
____ 24 push-ups (regular or modified)
____ 24 floors on stepper

DAY 140

____ *5-10 minute warm-up*
____ Fun Workout!*

Aerobics 530	Backpacking 570	Badminton 370
Raking leaves 330	Dancing 450	Basketball 490
Boating 210	Boxing 735	Bowling 245
Canoeing 570	Fishing 250	Frisbee 250
Gardening 330	Golfing 370	Horseback riding 330
Ice skating 570	Mowing lawn 450	Racquetball 570
Soccer 570	Swimming laps 650	Tennis 570
Volleyball 430	Walking (moderate) 300	

Own activity: _____
Duration: _____

*Average calories burned in one hour by a 180-pound person are shown. (http://www.nutristrategy.com/activitylist4.htm)

"Failure is impossible."—Susan B. Anthony

DAY 141
___ *5-10 minute warm-up*
___ 1 mile on recumbent bike
___ 15 floors on stepper
___ 1 mile on treadmill
___ 3 minutes on upright bike
___ 1 mile on recumbent bike
___ Rest 1-2 minutes

___ 25 floors on stepper
___ 0.25 mile on treadmill
___ 3 minutes on upright bike
___ 1 mile on recumbent bike
___ 0.25 mile on treadmill

DAY 142
___ *5-10 minute warm-up*
___ 1 mile on elliptical
___ 1 mile on Cybex arc trainer
___ 38 floors on stepper
___ 39 jumping jacks
___ 40 jump-rope revolutions
___ 41 floors on stepper
___ 42 jumping jacks

"Man is what he believes."—Anton Chekhov

DAY 143

____ *5-10 minute warm-up*
____ 5 minutes on treadmill
____ 2 minutes on recumbent bike
____ 5 minutes on treadmill, incline of "8"
____ 3 minutes on recumbent bike, level "8"
____ Rest 1-2 minutes

____ 5 minutes on treadmill, incline of "5"
____ 2 minutes on treadmill
____ 5 minutes on recumbent bike
____ 3 minutes on treadmill, incline of "2"

DAY 144

____ *5-10 minute warm-up*
____ 0.5 mile on elliptical
____ 15 floors on stepper
____ 1 mile on upright bike
____ 0.5 mile on elliptical
____ Rest 1-2 minutes

____ 0.5 mile on elliptical
____ 15 floors on stepper
____ 1 mile on upright bike
____ 0.5 mile on elliptical

"Our visions begin with our desires."—Audre Lorde

DAY 145

____ *5-10 minute warm-up*
____ 5 floors on stepper
____ 4 minutes on recumbent bike
____ 3 minutes on treadmill, incline of "12"
____ 2 minutes of jump rope
____ 1 mile on upright bike
____ Rest 1-2 minutes

____ 5 floors on stepper
____ 4 minutes on recumbent bike
____ 3 minutes on treadmill, incline of "8"
____ 2 minutes of jump rope
____ 1 mile on upright bike

DAY 146

____ *5-10 minute warm-up*
____ 11 minutes on Cybex arc trainer
____ 2 miles on recumbent bike
____ 50 jumping jacks
____ 11 minutes on Cybex arc trainer
____ 2 miles on recumbent bike
____ 50 jumping jacks
____ 11 push-ups (regular or modified)

"Instead of thinking about where you are, think about where you want to be."—Diana Rankin

DAY 147

____ *5-10 minute warm-up*
____ 0.5 mile on elliptical, level "5"
____ 10 floors on stepper
____ 0.5 mile on elliptical
____ Rest 1-2 minutes

____ 10 floors on stepper
____ 0.5 mile on treadmill, incline of "5"
____ 10 floors on stepper
____ 0.5 mile on treadmill, incline of "5"

DAY 148

____ *5-10 minute warm-up*
____ 175 jump-rope revolutions (rest when needed)
____ 1.75 miles on recumbent bike
____ 1.75 miles on upright bike, level "7"
____ 1.75 miles on upright bike
____ Rest 1-2 minutes

____ 175 jump-rope revolutions (rest when needed)
____ 0.75 mile on recumbent bike
____ 0.75 mile on upright bike, level "5"
____ 0.75 mile on upright bike

"Pain is never permanent."—Saint Teresa of Avila

DAY 149

____ *5-10 minute warm-up*
____ 5 minutes on elliptical
____ 4 minutes on treadmill
____ 2 minutes on treadmill, incline of "8"
____ 3 minutes on treadmill
____ 1 minute on treadmill, incline of "3"
____ Rest 1-2 minutes

____ 5 minutes on elliptical
____ 4 minutes on elliptical, level "6"
____ 3 minutes on elliptical
____ 2 minutes on elliptical, level "6"
____ 1 mile on Cybex arc trainer

DAY 150

____ *5-10 minute warm-up*
____ 55 jump-rope revolutions
____ 1.5 miles on upright bike
____ 55 jump-rope revolutions
____ 1.5 miles on recumbent bike
____ 55 jump-rope revolutions
____ 0.5 mile on Cybex arc trainer
____ Rest 1-2 minutes

____ 55 jump-rope revolutions
____ 1.5 miles on recumbent bike
____ 55 jump-rope revolutions
____ 1.5 miles on upright bike
____ 55 jump-rope revolutions
____ 1.5 miles on recumbent bike
____ 55 jump-rope revolutions
____ 0.5 mile on Cybex arc trainer

"Goals are dreams with deadlines."—Diana Scharf Hunt

DAY 151

____ *5-10 minute warm-up*
____ 1 minute on treadmill (walk)
____ 1 minute on treadmill (jog/run)
____ Repeat for 9 minutes

____ 2 miles on upright bike
____ 2 miles on recumbent bike
____ Rest 1-2 minutes

____ 1 minute on treadmill (walk)
____ 1 minute on treadmill (jog/run)
____ Repeat for 9 minutes

DAY 152

____ *5-10 minute warm-up*
____ 45 jump-rope revolutions
____ 4 minutes on treadmill
____ 2 miles on recumbent bike
____ 4 minutes on elliptical
____ 2 miles on recumbent bike
____ 45 jump-rope revolutions
____ Rest 1-2 minutes

____ 4 minutes on treadmill
____ 1 mile on recumbent bike
____ 4 minutes on elliptical
____ 1 mile on recumbent bike
____ 145 jump-rope revolutions (rest when needed)

"Courage doesn't always roar. Sometimes courage is the quiet voice at the end of the day saying, 'I will try again tomorrow.'"—Mary Anne Radmacher

DAY 153

____ *5-10 minute warm-up*
____ 3 minutes on treadmill, incline of "2"
____ 3 minutes on upright bike, level "12"
____ 3 minutes on treadmill, incline of "4"
____ 3 minutes on upright bike, level "4"
____ 3 minutes on treadmill, incline of "6"
____ 3 minutes on upright bike, level "12"
____ 3 minutes on treadmill, incline of "2"
____ 3 minutes on upright bike, level "4"
____ 6 minutes on Cybex arc trainer

DAY 154

____ *5-10 minute warm-up*
____ 29 jumping jacks
____ 2.9 miles on recumbent bike
____ 29 jumping jacks
____ 2.9 miles on recumbent bike
____ 29 jumping jacks
____ 2.9 miles on recumbent bike
____ 29 jumping jacks

"You can easily judge the character of others by how they treat those who can do nothing for them or to them."—Malcolm S. Forbes

DAY 155
____ *5-10 minute warm-up*
____ 1 mile on treadmill
____ 0.25 mile on elliptical
____ 0.75 mile on treadmill
____ 0.5 mile on elliptical
____ 0.5 mile on treadmill
____ 0.75 mile on elliptical
____ 0.25 mile on treadmill
____ 1 mile on elliptical

DAY 156
____ *5-10 minute warm-up*
____ 3 minutes on treadmill
____ 8 floors on stepper
____ 3 miles on upright bike
____ 8 minutes on Cybex arc trainer
____ 3 minutes on elliptical
____ 8 jump-rope revolutions
____ 3 minutes on treadmill
____ 8 minutes on Cybex arc trainer
____ 38 push-ups (regular or modified, rest when needed)

"Your goal should be out of reach but not out of sight."—Anita DeFrantz

Day 157

____ 5-10 minute warm-up
____ 1 mile on upright bike
____ 5 minutes on stepper
____ 7 minutes on treadmill, incline of "5"
____ 5 minutes on stepper
____ 1 mile on upright bike
____ 7 minutes on treadmill

Day 158

____ 5-10 minute warm-up
____ 3 minutes on elliptical
____ 30 jump-rope revolutions
____ 4 minutes on recumbent bike
____ 40 jump-rope revolutions
____ 5 minutes on elliptical
____ 50 jump-rope revolutions
____ 6 minutes on recumbent bike
____ 60 jump-rope revolutions
____ 7 minutes on elliptical
____ 70 jump-rope revolutions
____ 8 minutes on elliptical
____ 80 jump-rope revolutions

"I have to exercise in the morning before my brain figures out what I'm doing."— Marsh Doble

DAY 159

____ *5-10 minute warm-up*
____ 1 minute on treadmill, incline of "1"
____ 2 minutes on treadmill, incline of "2"
____ 3 minutes on treadmill, incline of "3"
____ 5 minutes on treadmill, incline of "5"
____ 6 minutes on treadmill, incline of "6"
____ 7 minutes on treadmill, incline of "7"
____ 8 minutes on treadmill, incline of "8"

DAY 160

____ *5-10 minute warm-up*
____ Fun Workout!*

Aerobics 530	Backpacking 570	Badminton 370
Raking leaves 330	Dancing 450	Basketball 490
Boating 210	Boxing 735	Bowling 245
Canoeing 570	Fishing 250	Frisbee 250
Gardening 330	Golfing 370	Horseback riding 330
Ice skating 570	Mowing lawn 450	Racquetball 570
Soccer 570	Swimming laps 650	Tennis 570
Volleyball 430	Walking (moderate) 300	

Own activity: _____
Duration: _____

*Average calories burned in one hour by a 180-pound person are shown. (http://www.nutristrategy.com/activitylist4.htm)

"Every second is of infinite value."—Johann Wolfgang von Goethe

DAY 161

____ *5-10 minute warm-up*
____ 2 miles on upright bike
____ 2 miles on recumbent bike
____ 8 minutes on treadmill
____ 2 miles on upright bike
____ 2 miles on recumbent bike

DAY 162

____ *5-10 minute warm-up*
____ 2 minutes on stepper
____ 3 minutes on treadmill, incline of "2"
____ 2 miles on recumbent bike
____ 4 minutes on stepper
____ 6 minutes on elliptical
____ 8 minutes on Cybex arc trainer

"I love the challenge of starting at zero every day and seeing how much I can accomplish."—Martha Stewart

DAY 163

___ *5-10 minute warm-up*
___ 30 jump-rope revolutions
___ 5 minutes on treadmill, incline of "3"
___ 27 jump-rope revolutions
___ 5 minutes on upright bike, level "3"
___ Rest 1-2 minutes

___ 24 jump-rope revolutions
___ 4 minutes on treadmill, incline of "2"
___ 21 jump-rope revolutions
___ 4 minutes on upright bike, level "2"
___ Rest 1-2 minutes

___ 18 jump-rope revolutions
___ 3 minutes on treadmill, incline of "3"
___ 15 jump-rope revolutions
___ 3 minutes on upright bike, level "2"

DAY 164

___ *5-10 minute warm-up*
___ 3 minutes on Cybex arc trainer
___ 60 jumping jacks
___ 0.5 mile on treadmill
___ 3 minutes on stepper
___ 60 jumping jacks
___ Rest 1-2 minutes

___ 3 minutes on Cybex arc trainer
___ 60 jumping jacks
___ 0.5 mile on treadmill
___ 3 minutes on stepper
___ 60 jumping jacks

"Energy is equal to desire and purpose."—Sheryl Adams

DAY 165
____ *5-10 minute warm-up*
____ 2 miles on Cybex arc trainer
____ 10 minutes on upright bike
____ 20 floors on stepper

DAY 166
____ *5-10 minute warm-up*
____ 6 minutes on treadmill
____ 6 minutes on recumbent bike
____ 7 minutes on treadmill, incline of "6"
____ 7 minutes on recumbent bike
____ 80 jumping jacks
____ 80 jump-rope revolutions
____ 9 push-ups (regular or modified)
____ 9 floors on stepper

*Remember to stay in your Target-Heart-Rate zone.

"You can have anything you want if you want it desperately enough. You must want it with an inner exuberance that erupts through the skin and joins the energy that created the world."—Sheila Graham

Day 167

____ *5-10 minute warm-up*
____ 20 floors on stepper
____ 1 mile on elliptical
____ 20 floors on stepper
____ 2 miles on recumbent bike
____ 20 floors on stepper
____ Rest 1-2 minutes

____ 1 mile on elliptical
____ 20 floors on stepper
____ 4 miles on recumbent bike
____ 20 floors on stepper
____ Rest 1-2 minutes

Day 168

____ *5-10 minute warm-up*
____ 10 minutes on recumbent bike
____ 100 jumping jacks
____ Rest 1-2 minutes

____ 8 minutes on Cybex arc trainer
____ 88 jumping jacks
____ 6 minutes on recumbent bike
____ 66 jumping jacks
____ Rest 1-2 minutes

____ 4 minutes on Cybex arc trainer
____ 44 jumping jacks
____ 2 minutes on recumbent bike
____ 22 jumping jacks

"The future is the most expensive luxury in the world."—Thornton Wilder

DAY 169

___ *5-10 minute warm-up*
___ 0.25 mile on treadmill
___ 25 jump-rope revolutions
___ 2.25 miles on upright bike
___ 25 jump-rope revolutions
___ Rest 1-2 minutes

___ 0.25 mile on treadmill
___ 25 jump-rope revolutions
___ 2.25 miles on upright bike
___ 25 jump-rope revolutions
___ Rest 1-2 minutes

___ 0.25 mile on treadmill
___ 25 jump-rope revolutions
___ 2.25 miles on upright bike
___ 25 jump-rope revolutions
___ Rest 1-2 minutes

DAY 170

___ *5-10 minute warm-up*
___ 3 minutes on elliptical
___ 1 mile on recumbent bike
___ 0.5 mile on elliptical
___ 3 minutes on recumbent bike, level "3"
___ Rest 1-2 minutes

___ 3 minutes on elliptical
___ 1 mile on recumbent bike
___ 0.5 mile on elliptical
___ 3 minutes on recumbent bike, level "3"
___ 6 minutes on treadmill

"Fatigue is the best pillow."—Benjamin Franklin

DAY 171

____ *5-10 minute warm-up*
____ 17 floors on stepper
____ 4 minutes on Cybex arc trainer
____ 17 jumping jacks
____ 4 minutes on treadmill, incline of "7"
____ Rest 1-2 minutes

____ 17 floors on stepper
____ 4 minutes on Cybex arc trainer
____ 17 jumping jacks
____ 4 minutes on treadmill, incline of "4"
____ 2 miles on upright bike

DAY 172

____ *5-10 minute warm-up*
____ 5 minutes on elliptical
____ 5 minutes on recumbent bike
____ 70 jump-rope revolutions
____ 7 minutes on recumbent bike
____ 3 minutes on elliptical
____ 7 minutes on treadmill, incline of "3"
____ 4 minutes on recumbent bike

"Put yourself in competition with yourself each day. Each morning look back upon your work of yesterday and then try to beat it."—Charles M. Sheldon

Day 173
___ *5-10 minute warm-up*
___ 30 jump-rope revolutions
___ 1 mile on treadmill
___ 30 jump-rope revolutions
___ 1 mile on Cybex arc trainer
___ Rest 1-2 minutes

___ 30 jump-rope revolutions
___ 0.5 mile on treadmill
___ 30 jump-rope revolutions
___ 0.5 mile on Cybex arc trainer
___ 30 jump-rope revolutions

Day 174
___ *5-10 minute warm-up*
___ 1 minute on treadmill (walk)
___ 1 minute on treadmill (jog/run)
___ Repeat for 17 minutes

___ 1 mile on recumbent bike, level "4"
___ 4 minutes on stepper
___ Rest 1-2 minutes

___ 1 minute on treadmill (walk)
___ 1 minute on treadmill (jog/run)
___ Repeat for 7 minutes

"Life is like a mirror. Smile at it, and it smiles back at you."—Peace Pilgrim

DAY 175

____ *5-10 minute warm-up*
____ 96 jump-rope revolutions
____ 9 minutes on treadmill, incline of "6"
____ 6 minutes on treadmill, incline of "9"
____ 96 jump-rope revolutions
____ Rest 1-2 minutes

____ 69 jump-rope revolutions
____ 6 minutes on treadmill, incline of "9"
____ 9 minutes on treadmill, incline of "6"
____ 69 jump-rope revolutions

DAY 176

____ *5-10 minute warm-up*
____ 7 minutes on Cybex arc trainer
____ 10 floors on stepper
____ 1.7 miles on upright bike
____ 6 minutes on Cybex arc trainer
____ 10 floors on stepper
____ 1.6 miles on upright bike
____ Rest 1-2 minutes

____ 5 minutes on Cybex arc trainer
____ 10 floors on stepper
____ 1.5 miles on upright bike
____ 4 minutes on Cybex arc trainer
____ 10 floors on stepper
____ 1.4 miles on upright bike

"The past cannot be changed. The future is yet in your power."—Mary Pickford

DAY 177
____ 5-10 minute warm-up
____ 70 jumping jacks
____ 7 minutes on treadmill, incline of "7"
____ 60 jumping jacks
____ 6 minutes on treadmill, incline of "6"
____ 50 jumping jacks
____ 5 minutes on treadmill, incline of "5"
____ 40 jumping jacks
____ 4 minutes on treadmill, incline of "4"
____ 30 jumping jacks
____ 3 minutes on treadmill, incline of "3"
____ 20 jumping jacks
____ 2 minutes on treadmill, incline of "2"
____ 10 jumping jacks
____ 1 minute on treadmill, incline of "10"

DAY 178
____ 5-10 minute warm-up
____ 4 minutes on Cybex arc trainer
____ 4 minutes on recumbent bike
____ 4 minutes on treadmill
____ 4 minutes on stepper
____ 4 minutes on elliptical
____ 4 minutes of jump rope
____ 4 minutes on treadmill

"I may not be there yet, but I am closer than I was yesterday"—José N. Harris.

DAY 179

____ *5-10 minute warm-up*
____ 6 minutes on Cybex arc trainer
____ 3 minutes on upright bike
____ 6 minutes on recumbent bike
____ 3 minutes on Cybex arc trainer
____ 6 minutes on upright bike, level "6"
____ 3 minutes on recumbent bike
____ 6 minutes on Cybex arc trainer

DAY 180

____ *5-10 minute warm-up*
____ Complete a 5K/10K race or (3.1/6.2 miles) on treadmill

Record your time: _____

"There's a difference between interest and commitment. When you're interested in doing something, you do it only when it's convenient. When you're committed to something, you accept no excuses, only results."—Kenneth Blanchard

DAY 181
____ *5-10 minute warm-up*
____ Fun Workout!*

Aerobics 530	Backpacking 570	Badminton 370
Raking leaves 330	Dancing 450	Basketball 490
Boating 210	Boxing 735	Bowling 245
Canoeing 570	Fishing 250	Frisbee 250
Gardening 330	Golfing 370	Horseback riding 330
Ice skating 570	Mowing lawn 450	Racquetball 570
Soccer 570	Swimming laps 650	Tennis 570
Volleyball 430	Walking (moderate) 300	

Own activity: _____
Duration: _____

*Average calories burned in one hour by a 180-pound person are shown. (http://www.nutristrategy.com/activitylist4.htm)

DAY 182
____ *5-10 minute warm-up*
____ 19 floors on stepper
____ 1 mile on treadmill
____ 9 floors on stepper
____ 1 mile on elliptical
____ 9 floors on stepper
____ 19 floors on stepper

"When we are no longer able to change a situation, we are challenged to change ourselves."—Viktor E. Frankl

DAY 183

___ *5-10 minute warm-up*
___ 2 minutes on treadmill (jog/run)
___ 1 minute on treadmill (walk)
___ Repeat for 22 minutes

___ 1 mile on upright bike
___ 4 minutes on recumbent bike
___ 14 push-ups (regular or modified)

DAY 184

___ *5-10 minute warm-up*
___ 22 jumping jacks
___ 4 minutes on upright bike
___ 20 jumping jacks
___ 4 minutes on recumbent bike
___ 18 jumping jacks
___ 4 minutes on elliptical
___ 16 jumping jacks
___ 4 minutes on upright bike
___ 14 jumping jacks
___ 4 minutes on recumbent bike
___ 12 jumping jacks
___ 4 minutes on elliptical
___ 10 jumping jacks

"Change before you have to."—Jack Welch

DAY 185

____ 5-10 minute warm-up
____ 7 minutes on treadmill
____ 9 minutes on upright bike
____ 8 minutes on stepper
____ 6 minutes on treadmill
____ 5 minutes on upright bike

DAY 186

____ 5-10 minute warm-up
____ 1 minute of jump rope
____ 1 mile on recumbent bike
____ 1 minute of jump rope
____ 1 mile on upright bike

____ Repeat above grouping 4 times

*Remember to stay in your Target-Heart-Rate zone.

"I tried every diet in the book. I tried some that weren't in the book. I tried eating the book. It tasted better than most of the diets."—Dolly Parton

DAY 187

____ *5-10 minute warm-up*
____ 0.5 mile on treadmill
____ 0.5 mile on Cybex arc trainer
____ 5 minutes on recumbent bike
____ Rest 1-2 minutes

____ 0.5 mile on treadmill, incline of "5"
____ 0.5 mile on Cybex arc, level "5"
____ 5 minutes on recumbent bike
____ 0.5 mile on treadmill

DAY 188

____ *5-10 minute warm-up*
____ 2 minutes on elliptical
____ 4 minutes on treadmill, incline of "4"
____ 6 minutes on upright bike
____ 8 floors on stepper
____ 10 jump-rope revolutions
____ Rest 1-2 minutes

____ 3 minutes on elliptical
____ 5 minutes on treadmill, incline of "5"
____ 7 minutes on upright bike
____ 9 floors on stepper
____ 11 jump-rope revolutions

"I like long walks, especially when they are taken by people who annoy me."—Fred Allen

DAY 189

___ *5-10 minute warm-up*
___ 1 mile on recumbent bike
___ 0.5 mile on treadmill
___ 0.5 mile on Cybex arc trainer
___ 1 mile on treadmill
___ 0.5 mile on recumbent bike
___ 0.5 mile on Cybex arc trainer
___ 2 miles on recumbent bike

DAY 190

___ *5-10 minute warm-up*
___ 3 minutes on elliptical
___ 6 minutes on recumbent bike, level "6"
___ 11 minutes on upright bike
___ Rest 1-2 minutes

___ 25 push-ups (regular or modified)
___ 3 minutes on recumbent bike, level "3"
___ 6 minutes on elliptical
___ 11 floors on stepper

"Change does not roll in on the wheels of inevitability, but comes through continuous struggle."—Martin Luther King, Jr.

DAY 191
____ *5-10 minute warm-up*
____ 2 minutes on treadmill, incline of "8"
____ 28 jump-rope revolutions
____ 8 minutes on treadmill, incline of "2"
____ 82 jumping jacks
____ 1 mile on recumbent bike
____ 14 floors on stepper
____ 14 minutes on treadmill

DAY 192
____ *5-10 minute warm-up*
____ 50 jumping jacks
____ 0.5 mile on elliptical
____ 0.5 mile on Cybex arc trainer
____ Rest 1-2 minutes

____ 50 jumping jacks
____ 0.5 mile on elliptical
____ 0.5 mile on Cybex arc trainer
____ 9 minutes on upright bike, level "5"
____ 90 jumping jacks

"Today I will do what others won't, so tomorrow I can accomplish what others can't."—Jerry Rice

Day 193
____ *5-10 minute warm-up*
____ 7 minutes on treadmill
____ 4 minutes on stepper
____ 8 minutes on recumbent bike
____ 4 minutes on treadmill
____ 7 minutes on recumbent bike
____ 4 minutes on stepper

Day 194
____ *5-10 minute warm-up*
____ 20 jump-rope revolutions
____ 5 minutes on elliptical
____ 30 jump-rope revolutions
____ 5 minutes on elliptical
____ 10 minutes on treadmill
____ 20 jump-rope revolutions
____ 6 minutes on elliptical
____ 30 jump-rope revolutions
____ 5 minutes on elliptical

"Keep things consistent and you'll turn any health goal into an automatic (and eventually unconscious) behavior."—Yuri Elkaim

DAY 195

___ *5-10 minute warm-up*
___ 60 jumping jacks
___ 2 minutes on Cybex arc trainer
___ 5 minutes on upright bike
___ Rest 1-2 minutes

___ 60 jumping jacks
___ 0.5 mile on Cybex arc trainer
___ 2 miles on upright bike
___ Rest 1-2 minutes

___ 60 jumping jacks
___ 1 mile on Cybex arc trainer
___ 3 miles on upright bike

DAY 196

___ *5-10 minute warm-up*
___ 2 miles on recumbent bike
___ 11 floors on stepper
___ 20 jump-rope revolutions
___ 10 minutes on treadmill, incline of "3"
___ 6 minutes on elliptical, level "3"
___ 30 floors on stepper

"Of course, I want to be number one. But being happy and healthy is the most important thing."—Venus Williams

DAY 197

____ *5-10 minute warm-up*
____ 1 minute on treadmill (walk)
____ 1 minute on treadmill (jog/run)
____ Repeat for 12 minutes

____ 30 push-ups (regular or modified)
____ 3 minutes on recumbent bike
____ 3 minutes on upright bike
____ 3 minutes on recumbent bike, level "3"
____ 3 minutes on upright bike
____ 6 minutes on treadmill, incline of "6"

DAY 198

____ *5-10 minute warm-up*
____ 30 jump-rope revolutions
____ 12 minutes on elliptical
____ 120 jump-rope revolutions
____ 12 minutes on Cybex arc trainer
____ 60 jump-rope revolutions
____ 12 minutes on elliptical

"Happiness always looks small while you hold it in your hands, but let it go, and you learn at once how big and precious it is."—Maxim Gorky

DAY 199

____ *5-10 minute warm-up*
____ 1 minute on treadmill (walk)
____ 1 minute on treadmill (jog/run)
____ Repeat for 10 minutes

____ 2.5 miles on recumbent bike
____ 25 jump-rope revolutions

____ 1 minute on treadmill (walk)
____ 1 minute on treadmill (jog/run)
____ Repeat for 10 minutes

DAY 200

____ *5-10 minute warm-up*
____ Fun Workout!*

Aerobics 530	Backpacking 570	Badminton 370
Raking leaves 330	Dancing 450	Basketball 490
Boating 210	Boxing 735	Bowling 245
Canoeing 570	Fishing 250	Frisbee 250
Gardening 330	Golfing 370	Horseback riding 330
Ice skating 570	Mowing lawn 450	Racquetball 570
Soccer 570	Swimming laps 650	Tennis 570
Volleyball 430	Walking (moderate) 300	

Own activity: _____
Duration: _____

*Average calories burned in one hour by a 180-pound person are shown. (http://www.nutristrategy.com/activitylist4.htm)

"It's not about being the best; it's about being better than you were yesterday."—Anonymous

Day 201

____ *5-10 minute warm-up*

____ 1 mile on recumbent bike

____ 11 minutes on Cybex arc trainer

____ 2 minutes on treadmill, incline of "12"

____ 12 jump-rope revolutions

____ 3 minutes on Cybex arc trainer

____ 13 jumping jacks

____ 4 minutes on treadmill, incline of "13"

____ 14 floors on stepper

Day 202

____ *5-10 minute warm-up*

____ 2 minutes on elliptical

____ 4 minutes on upright bike, level "4"

____ 4 minutes on elliptical

____ 6 minutes on upright bike, level "6"

____ 6 minutes on elliptical

____ 8 minutes on upright bike, level "8"

"Never let the odds keep you from doing what you know in your heart you were meant to do."—H. Jackson Brown, Jr.

DAY 203

____ *5-10 minute warm-up*
____ 7 minutes on treadmill
____ 6 minutes on recumbent bike
____ 3 minutes on treadmill, incline of "6"
____ 5 minutes on upright bike
____ 9 floors on stepper
____ 1 mile on recumbent bike
____ 5 minutes on treadmill, incline of "5"

DAY 204

____ *5-10 minute warm-up*
____ 8 minutes on Cybex arc trainer
____ 8 minutes on treadmill
____ 6 minutes on Cybex arc trainer
____ 2 minutes on stepper
____ 3 minutes on treadmill, incline of "3"
____ 1 mile on upright bike

*Remember to stay in your Target-Heart-Rate zone.

"Don't be afraid to take a big step if one is indicated. You can't cross a chasm in two small jumps."—David Lloyd George

DAY 205

___ *5-10 minute warm-up*
___ 3 minutes on recumbent bike
___ 3 minutes of jump rope
___ 6 minutes on elliptical
___ 6 minutes on recumbent bike
___ 6 minutes on elliptical
___ 3 minutes of jump rope
___ 3 minutes on recumbent bike

DAY 206

___ *5-10 minute warm-up*
___ 10 floors on stepper
___ 10 minutes on treadmill
___ 20 floors on stepper
___ 2 minutes of jumping jacks
___ 25 push-ups (regular or modified)
___ 8 minutes on treadmill, incline of "2"
___ 10 floors on stepper
___ 2 minutes of jumping jacks
___ 4 minutes on treadmill, incline of "4"

"Keep your promises to yourself."—David Harold Fink

DAY 207

____ *5-10 minute warm-up*
____ 50 jumping jacks
____ 50 jump-rope revolutions
____ 0.5 mile on Cybex arc trainer
____ 1 mile on upright bike
____ Rest 1-2 minutes

____ 50 jumping jacks
____ 50 jump-rope revolutions
____ 0.5 mile on Cybex arc trainer
____ 1 mile upright bike
____ Rest 1-2 minutes

____ 50 jumping jacks
____ 50 jump-rope revolutions
____ 0.5 mile on Cybex arc trainer
____ 1 mile upright bike

DAY 208

____ *5-10 minute warm-up*
____ 2 minutes on treadmill
____ 1 mile on recumbent bike
____ 0.5 mile on treadmill
____ 2 minutes on stepper
____ 3 minutes on upright bike
____ Rest 1-2 minutes

____ 2 minutes on treadmill, incline of "2"
____ 1 mile on recumbent bike
____ 0.5 mile on treadmill
____ 2 minutes on stepper
____ 3 minutes on upright bike, level "3"

"Arriving at one goal is the starting point to another."—John Dewey

DAY 209

____ *5-10 minute warm-up*
____ 60 jumping jacks
____ 1 mile on upright bike
____ 0.5 mile on elliptical
____ 2 miles on upright bike
____ 0.75 mile on elliptical
____ 60 jumping jacks
____ 0.5 mile on elliptical
____ 3 miles on upright bike
____ 0.5 mile on elliptical
____ 60 jumping jacks

DAY 210

____ *5-10 minute warm-up*
____ 6 minutes on treadmill, incline of "2"
____ 2 minutes on stepper
____ 2 minutes on upright bike
____ 9 minutes on treadmill
____ 4 minutes on stepper
____ 8 minutes on upright bike

"Set short-term goals, and you'll win games. Set long-term goals, and you'll win championships."—Joe Paterno

DAY 211

____ *5-10 minute warm-up*
____ 3 minutes on recumbent bike
____ 1 mile on Cybex arc trainer
____ 6 minutes on elliptical
____ 1 mile on Cybex arc trainer
____ 9 minutes on elliptical
____ 1 mile on recumbent bike

DAY 212

____ *5-10 minute warm-up*
____ 7 minutes on treadmill, incline of "4"
____ 4 miles on upright bike
____ 5 minutes on stepper
____ 4 minutes on treadmill
____ 1 mile on recumbent bike
____ 5 minutes on stepper

"Everything's in the mind. That's where it all starts. Knowing what you want is the first step toward getting it."—Mae West

Day 213
____ *5-10 minute warm-up*
____ 60 jumping jacks
____ 6 minutes on Cybex arc trainer
____ 4 minutes on recumbent bike
____ 40 jump-rope revolutions
____ 50 jumping jacks
____ 5 minutes on Cybex arc trainer
____ 3 minutes on recumbent bike
____ 40 jump-rope revolutions
____ 1 mile on elliptical

Day 214
____ *5-10 minute warm-up*
____ 0.75 mile on treadmill
____ 20 floors on stepper
____ 0.75 mile on treadmill, incline of "2"
____ 15 floors on stepper
____ 0.5 mile on treadmill, incline of "5"
____ 10 floors on stepper
____ 0.5 mile on treadmill, incline of "1"
____ 8 floors on stepper
____ 0.25 mile on treadmill, incline of "8"
____ 5 floors on stepper
____ 0.25 mile on treadmill, incline of "5"

"Clear your mind of can't."—Samuel Johnson

DAY 215

____ *5-10 minute warm-up*
____ 10 minutes on upright bike
____ 10 minutes on elliptical
____ 10 minutes on treadmill

DAY 216

____ *5-10 minute warm-up*
____ 0.5 mile on Cybex arc trainer
____ 30 jumping jacks
____ 3 minutes on treadmill
____ 30 jump-rope revolutions
____ Rest 1-2 minutes

____ 60 jumping jacks
____ 6 minutes on treadmill
____ 60 jump-rope revolutions
____ Rest 1-2 minutes

____ 90 jumping jacks
____ 9 minutes on treadmill
____ 90 jump-rope revolutions
____ 0.5 mile on Cybex arc trainer

"Old minds are like old horses; you must exercise them if you wish to keep them in working order."—John Adams

DAY 217

____ *5-10 minute warm-up*
____ 7 minutes on elliptical
____ 2 miles on recumbent bike
____ 6 minutes on treadmill, incline of "6"
____ 4 minutes on elliptical
____ 8 floors on stepper
____ 6 minutes on recumbent bike

DAY 218

____ *5-10 minute warm-up*
____ 0.25 mile on treadmill
____ 0.25 mile on Cybex arc trainer
____ 25 jump-rope revolutions
____ 25 floors on stepper
____ 25 jumping jacks
____ 0.25 mile on treadmill
____ 0.25 mile on Cybex arc trainer
____ Rest 1-2 minutes

____ 25 jump-rope revolutions
____ 25 floors on stepper
____ 25 jumping jacks
____ 0.25 mile on treadmill
____ 0.25 mile on Cybex arc trainer
____ 25 jump-rope revolutions
____ 25 floors on stepper
____ 25 jumping jacks

"Obstacles are those frightful things you see when you take your eyes off the goal."—Henry Ford

DAY 219

____ *5-10 minute warm-up*
____ 2 miles on upright bike
____ 1 mile on elliptical
____ 9 minutes on recumbent bike, level "9"
____ 1 mile on upright bike
____ 2 minutes on elliptical

DAY 220

____ *5-10 minute warm-up*
____ Fun Workout!*

Aerobics 530	Backpacking 570	Badminton 370
Raking leaves 330	Dancing 450	Basketball 490
Boating 210	Boxing 735	Bowling 245
Canoeing 570	Fishing 250	Frisbee 250
Gardening 330	Golfing 370	Horseback riding 330
Ice skating 570	Mowing lawn 450	Racquetball 570
Soccer 570	Swimming laps 650	Tennis 570
Volleyball 430	Walking (moderate) 300	

Own activity: _____
Duration: _____

*Average calories burned in one hour by a 180-pound person are shown. (http://www.nutristrategy.com/activitylist4.htm)

"No one knows what he can do until he tries."—Publilius Syrus

DAY 221
____ *5-10 minute warm-up*
____ 3 minutes on elliptical
____ 9 minutes on upright bike
____ 9 jump-rope revolutions
____ 1 mile on upright bike
____ 1 mile on elliptical
____ 2 miles on upright bike
____ 99 jump-rope revolutions

DAY 222
____ *5-10 minute warm-up*
____ 8 minutes of jump rope (rest when needed)
____ 2 minutes on recumbent bike
____ 2 minutes on upright bike, level "8"
____ 2 minutes on treadmill, incline of "8"
____ 2 miles on recumbent bike
____ 2 minutes on treadmill
____ 2 minutes on upright bike, level "2"
____ 6 minutes of jump rope (rest when needed)

"You don't have to be afraid of change. You don't have to worry about what's being taken away. Just look to see what's been added."—Jackie Greer

DAY 223

___ *5-10 minute warm-up*
___ 8 minutes on stepper
___ 2 miles on upright bike
___ 9 minutes on Cybex arc trainer
___ 1 mile on upright bike
___ 8 minutes on stepper

DAY 224

___ *5-10 minute warm-up*
___ 3 minutes on treadmill, incline of "9"
___ 9 minutes on elliptical
___ 8 minutes on treadmill, incline of "2"
___ 2 minutes of jump rope
___ 5 minutes on elliptical
___ 4 minutes on recumbent bike

"If one advances confidently in the direction of his dreams, and endeavors to live the life which he has imagined, he will meet with a success unexpected in common hours."—Henry David Thoreau

DAY 225

___ *5-10 minute warm-up*
___ Complete a 5K/10K race or (3.1/6.2 miles) on treadmill

Record your time: _____

DAY 226

___ *5-10 minute warm-up*
___ Fun Workout!*

Aerobics 530	Backpacking 570	Badminton 370
Raking leaves 330	Dancing 450	Basketball 490
Boating 210	Boxing 735	Bowling 245
Canoeing 570	Fishing 250	Frisbee 250
Gardening 330	Golfing 370	Horseback riding 330
Ice skating 570	Mowing lawn 450	Racquetball 570
Soccer 570	Swimming laps 650	Tennis 570
Volleyball 430	Walking (moderate) 300	

Own activity: _____
Duration: _____

*Average calories burned in one hour by a 180-pound person are shown. (http://www.nutristrategy.com/activitylist4.htm)

"Health is the vital principle of bliss."—James Thomson

DAY 227

____ *5-10 minute warm-up*
____ 1 minute on treadmill (walk)
____ 1 minute on treadmill (jog/run)
____ Repeat for 8 minutes
____ Rest 1-2 minutes

____ 4 minutes on upright bike
____ 1 minute on treadmill (walk)
____ 1 minute on treadmill (jog/run)
____ Repeat for 22 minutes

DAY 228

____ *5-10 minute warm-up*
____ 3 minutes on stepper
____ 3 minutes on treadmill
____ 0.5 mile on elliptical
____ 33 jumping jacks
____ 2 minutes on stepper
____ 2 minutes on treadmill, incline of "10"
____ Rest 1-2 minutes

____ 25 push-ups (regular or modified)
____ 0.5 mile on elliptical
____ 22 jumping jacks
____ 1 minute on stepper
____ 1 minute on treadmill, incline of "15"
____ 0.25 mile on elliptical
____ 11 jumping jacks

"One does not discover new lands without consenting to lose sight of the shore for a very long time."—Andre Gide

DAY 229
____ *5-10 minute warm-up*
____ 15 minutes on Cybex arc trainer
____ 5 minutes on upright bike
____ 10 minutes on Cybex arc trainer
____ 5 minutes on upright bike

DAY 230
____ *5-10 minute warm-up*
____ 15 floors on stepper
____ 0.5 mile on treadmill
____ 12 floors on stepper
____ 0.5 mile on treadmill
____ 9 floors on stepper
____ 0.5 mile on treadmill
____ 7 floors on stepper
____ 5 minutes on treadmill

"Start by doing what's necessary; then do what's possible, and suddenly you are doing the impossible."—Saint Francis of Assisi

DAY 231

___ *5-10 minute warm-up*
___ 9 minutes on upright bike
___ 1 mile on recumbent bike, level "9"
___ 9 minutes on elliptical
___ 1 mile on upright bike
___ 6 minutes on recumbent bike
___ 4 minutes on elliptical
___ 12 jumping jacks
___ 20 jump-rope revolutions

DAY 232

___ *5-10 minute warm-up*
___ 1 mile on Cybex arc trainer
___ 4 minutes on upright bike
___ 9 minutes on treadmill
___ 16 jump-rope revolutions
___ 25 jumping jacks
___ 36 floors on stepper
___ 49 jump-rope revolutions
___ 64 jumping jacks
___ 81 jump-rope revolutions
___ 100 jumping jacks

"Each day comes bearing its own gifts. Untie the ribbons."—Ruth Ann Schabacker

Day 233

____ *5-10 minute warm-up*
____ 8 minutes on elliptical
____ 7 minutes on recumbent bike
____ 6 minutes on upright bike, level "6"
____ 5 minutes on elliptical
____ 4 minutes on upright bike, level "4"
____ 3 minutes on recumbent bike
____ 2 minutes on treadmill, incline of "12"
____ 1 minute on recumbent bike, level "15"

Day 234

____ *5-10 minute warm-up*
____ 2 minutes on stepper
____ 3 minutes of jump rope (rest when needed)
____ 4 minutes on treadmill
____ 5 jumping jacks
____ 9 minutes on Cybex arc trainer
____ 4 minutes on treadmill, incline of "4"
____ 15 floors on stepper
____ 1 mile on Cybex arc trainer

"You have to set new goals everyday."—Julie Krone

DAY 235

____ *5-10 minute warm-up*
____ 1 mile on recumbent bike
____ 0.5 mile on elliptical
____ 0.25 mile on treadmill, incline of "2"
____ 0.5 mile on elliptical
____ 2 miles on upright bike
____ 0.5 mile on treadmill
____ 2 miles on upright bike
____ 0.5 mile on treadmill
____ 1 mile on recumbent bike
____ 0.5 mile on elliptical

DAY 236

____ *5-10 minute warm-up*
____ 7 minutes on stepper
____ 4 miles on recumbent bike
____ 3 minutes on treadmill, incline of "10"
____ 2 miles on recumbent bike
____ 6 floors on stepper
____ 32 jumping jacks

"That which does not kill us makes us stronger."—Friedrich Nietzsche

DAY 237

____ *5-10 minute warm-up*
____ 5 minutes on elliptical
____ 10 minutes on upright bike
____ 15 jump-rope revolutions
____ 20 floors on stepper
____ 25 jump-rope revolutions
____ 30 floors on stepper
____ 35 jump-rope revolutions
____ 40 floors on stepper
____ 5 minutes on elliptical

DAY 238

____ *5-10 minute warm-up*
____ 2 minutes on treadmill, incline of "15"
____ 3 minutes on treadmill, incline of "10"
____ 4 minutes on treadmill, incline of "5"
____ 5 minutes on upright bike, level "5"
____ 1.5 miles on Cybex arc trainer

*Remember to stay in your Target-Heart-Rate zone.

"We don't know who we are until we see what we can do."—Martha Grimes

DAY 239

___ *5-10 minute warm-up*
___ 100 jumping jacks
___ 5 minutes on elliptical
___ 25 push-ups (regular or modified)
___ 5 miles on recumbent bike
___ 100 jumping jacks

DAY 240

___ *5-10 minute warm-up*
___ Fun Workout!*

Aerobics 530	Backpacking 570	Badminton 370
Raking leaves 330	Dancing 450	Basketball 490
Boating 210	Boxing 735	Bowling 245
Canoeing 570	Fishing 250	Frisbee 250
Gardening 330	Golfing 370	Horseback riding 330
Ice skating 570	Mowing lawn 450	Racquetball 570
Soccer 570	Swimming laps 650	Tennis 570
Volleyball 430	Walking (moderate) 300	

Own activity: _____
Duration: _____

*Average calories burned in one hour by a 180-pound person are shown. (http://www.nutristrategy.com/activitylist4.htm)

"It is in changing that things find purpose."—Heraclitus.

Day 241
____ *5-10 minute warm-up*
____ 3 minutes on upright bike
____ 30 jumping jacks
____ 4 minutes on Cybex arc trainer
____ 40 jumping jacks
____ 5 minutes on elliptical
____ 50 jumping jacks
____ 6 minutes on upright bike
____ 60 jumping jacks
____ 7 minutes on Cybex arc trainer
____ 70 jumping jacks

Day 242
____ *5-10 minute warm-up*
____ 22 floors on stepper
____ 12 minutes on treadmill
____ 12 floors on stepper
____ 2 minutes on treadmill, incline of "12"
____ Rest 1-2 minutes

____ 25 push-ups (regular or modified)
____ 2 miles on upright bike
____ 2 minutes on treadmill
____ 2 miles on recumbent bike
____ 2 minutes on treadmill

"Being stuck is a position few of us like. We want something new but cannot let go of the old—old ideas, beliefs, habits, even thoughts. We are out of contact with our own genius. Sometimes we know we are stuck; sometimes we don't. In both cases we have to do something."
—Rush Limbaugh

Day 243
____ *5-10 minute warm-up*
____ 50 jump-rope revolutions
____ 0.5 mile on elliptical
____ 1.5 miles on upright bike
____ 50 jump-rope revolutions
____ 0.5 mile on treadmill, incline of "5"
____ 0.5 mile on elliptical
____ Rest 1-2 minutes

____ 50 jump-rope revolutions
____ 1.5 miles on upright bike
____ 0.5 mile on elliptical
____ 150 jump-rope revolutions
____ 5 minutes on treadmill

Day 244
____ *5-10 minute warm-up*
____ 15 floors on stepper
____ 14 jumping jacks
____ 13 floors on stepper
____ 12 jumping jacks
____ 11 minutes on treadmill
____ 10 floors on stepper
____ 9 jumping jacks
____ 8 minutes on Cybex arc trainer
____ 7 floors on stepper
____ 6 jumping jacks
____ 5 minutes on Cybex arc trainer
____ 4 floors on stepper
____ 3 minutes on treadmill
____ 2 floors on stepper
____ 1 minute on recumbent bike

"Bloom where you are planted."—Anonymous

Day 245

___ *5-10 minute warm-up*
___ 9 minutes on treadmill, incline of "11"
___ 11 minutes on upright bike, level "9"
___ 9 minutes on treadmill, incline of "9"
___ 11 jumping jacks

Day 246

___ *5-10 minute warm-up*
___ 8 minutes on elliptical, level "2"
___ 2 minutes on stepper
___ 8 minutes on recumbent bike
___ 2 minutes on stepper
___ 8 minutes on elliptical
___ 2 minutes on recumbent bike

*Remember to stay in your Target-Heart-Rate zone.

"'How does one become a butterfly?' she asked pensively.
'You must want to fly so much that you are willing to give up being a caterpillar.'"—Trina Paulus

DAY 247

____ *5-10 minute warm-up*
____ 15 floors on stepper
____ 1 mile on Cybex arc trainer
____ 1 mile on upright bike
____ 0.5 mile on Cybex arc trainer
____ 1 mile on upright bike
____ 25 push-ups (regular or modified)
____ 15 floors on stepper
____ 0.75 mile on Cybex arc trainer
____ 1 mile on upright bike
____ 0.5 mile on Cybex arc trainer
____ 0.75 mile on upright bike
____ 15 floors on stepper

DAY 248

____ *5-10 minute warm-up*
____ 7 minutes on treadmill
____ 45 jump-rope revolutions
____ 6 minutes on treadmill, incline of "4.5"
____ 40 jump-rope revolutions
____ 5 minutes on treadmill, incline of "4"
____ 35 jump-rope revolutions
____ 4 minutes on treadmill, incline of "3.5"
____ 30 jump-rope revolutions
____ 3 minutes on treadmill, incline of "3"
____ 25 jump-rope revolutions
____ 2 minutes on treadmill, incline of "2.5"
____ 20 jump-rope revolutions
____ 1 minute on treadmill, incline of "2"

"What's important is finding out what works for you."—Henry Moore

Day 249

____ *5-10 minute warm-up*
____ 1 mile on elliptical
____ 2 miles on recumbent bike
____ 1 mile on upright bike
____ 1 mile on Cybex arc trainer
____ 2 miles on recumbent bike
____ 1 mile on upright bike

Day 250

____ *5-10 minute warm-up*
____ 1 minute on treadmill (walk)
____ 1 minute on treadmill (jog/run)
____ Repeat for 16 minutes

____ 25 push-ups (regular or modified)
____ 4 minutes on upright bike
____ 1 mile on recumbent bike
____ Rest 1-2 minutes

____ 1 minute on treadmill (walk)
____ 1 minute on treadmill (jog/run)
____ Repeat for 12 minutes

"The only joy in the world is to begin."—Cesare Pavese

Day 251

___ *5-10 minute warm-up*
___ 60 jumping jacks
___ 8 minutes on Cybex arc trainer
___ 1 mile on recumbent bike
___ 4 minutes on Cybex arc trainer
___ 2 miles on recumbent bike
___ 8 minutes on elliptical
___ 60 jumping jacks

Day 252

___ *5-10 minute warm-up*
___ 2 minutes on stepper
___ 0.5 mile on treadmill
___ 5 miles on upright bike
___ 2 minutes on stepper
___ 0.5 mile on treadmill
___ 5 minutes on stepper

"'Stressed' spelled backwards is 'desserts.' Coincidence? I think not!"
—Anonymous

DAY 253

____ *5-10 minute warm-up*
____ 73 jump-rope revolutions
____ 7 minutes on elliptical
____ 3 minutes on recumbent bike
____ 73 jump-rope revolutions
____ 7 minutes on elliptical
____ 3 minutes on recumbent bike
____ 73 jump-rope revolutions
____ 7 minutes on elliptical
____ 3 minutes on treadmill

DAY 254

____ *5-10 minute warm-up*
____ 1 mile on Cybex arc trainer
____ 10 floors on stepper
____ 1 mile on upright bike
____ 10 floors on stepper
____ 1 mile on Cybex arc trainer
____ 10 floors on stepper
____ 1 mile on upright bike

"Everyone wants to live on top of the mountain, but all the happiness and growth occurs while you're climbing it."—Attributed to Andy Rooney

DAY 255

____ *5-10 minute warm-up*
____ 35 floors on stepper
____ 3.5 miles on recumbent bike
____ 3 minutes on treadmill, incline of "3.5"
____ 35 floors on stepper
____ 3.5 miles on recumbent bike
____ 3 minutes on treadmill, incline of "3.5"

DAY 256

____ *5-10 minute warm-up*
____ 0.5 mile on elliptical
____ 50 jumping jacks
____ 0.5 mile on Cybex arc trainer
____ 50 jumping jacks
____ 1 mile on recumbent bike
____ 50 jumping jacks
____ 11 minutes on upright bike
____ Rest 1-2 minutes

____ 25 push-ups (regular or modified)
____ 0.5 mile on elliptical
____ 50 jumping jacks
____ 0.5 mile on Cybex arc trainer
____ 50 jumping jacks
____ 1 mile on recumbent bike
____ 50 jumping jacks
____ 1 minute on upright bike

"If you spend your whole life waiting for the storm, you'll never enjoy the sunshine."—Morris West

DAY 257

____ *5-10 minute warm-up*
____ 6 minutes on treadmill, incline of "3"
____ 3 minutes on stepper
____ 8 minutes on treadmill
____ 5 minutes on recumbent bike
____ 2 minutes on stepper
____ 7 minutes on treadmill, incline of "2"

DAY 258

____ *5-10 minute warm-up*
____ 5 minutes on Cybex arc trainer
____ 8 minutes on upright bike
____ 8 minutes on Cybex arc trainer
____ 1 mile on upright bike
____ 1 mile on Cybex arc trainer
____ 2 miles on upright bike

"You have to stay in shape. My grandmother, she started walking five miles a day when she was sixty. She's ninety-seven today, and we don't know where the hell she is."—Ellen DeGeneres

DAY 259

____ *5-10 minute warm-up*
____ 1 mile on treadmill
____ 100 jump-rope revolutions
____ 2 miles on upright bike
____ 100 jump-rope revolutions
____ 1 mile on treadmill

DAY 260

____ *5-10 minute warm-up*
____ Fun Workout!*

Aerobics 530	Backpacking 570	Badminton 370
Raking leaves 330	Dancing 450	Basketball 490
Boating 210	Boxing 735	Bowling 245
Canoeing 570	Fishing 250	Frisbee 250
Gardening 330	Golfing 370	Horseback riding 330
Ice skating 570	Mowing lawn 450	Racquetball 570
Soccer 570	Swimming laps 650	Tennis 570
Volleyball 430	Walking (moderate) 300	

Own activity: _____

Duration: _____

*Average calories burned in one hour by a 180-pound person are shown. (http://www.nutristrategy.com/activitylist4.htm)

"Nothing tastes as good as being healthy feels."—Anonymous

DAY 261

____ *5-10 minute warm-up*
____ 1 minute on treadmill (walk)
____ 1 minute on treadmill (jog/run)
____ Repeat for 15 minutes

____ 2 miles on recumbent bike
____ 25 push-ups (regular or modified)
____ Rest 1-2 minutes

____ 1 minute on treadmill (walk)
____ 1 minute on treadmill (jog/run)
____ Repeat for 10 minutes

DAY 262

____ *5-10 minute warm-up*
____ 2 minutes on treadmill, incline of "3"
____ 3 minutes on stepper
____ 3 minutes on treadmill, incline of "4"
____ 4 minutes on recumbent bike
____ 9 minutes on treadmill, incline of "3"
____ 4 minutes on stepper
____ 7 minutes on treadmill, incline of "4"

"It's been my experience that you can nearly always enjoy things if you make up your mind firmly that you will."—L. M. Montgomery

DAY 263

____ *5-10 minute warm-up*
____ 0.5 mile on Cybex arc trainer
____ 2 miles on recumbent bike
____ 1 mile on Cybex arc trainer
____ 1 mile on upright bike
____ 2 miles on recumbent bike
____ 75 jump-rope revolutions
____ 0.5 mile on Cybex arc trainer

DAY 264

____ *5-10 minute warm-up*
____ 1 mile on elliptical
____ 45 jumping jacks
____ 4.5 miles on upright bike
____ 1 mile on elliptical
____ 45 jumping jacks

*Remember to stay in your Target-Heart-Rate zone.

"He who has health, has hope; and he who has hope, has everything."—Arabian proverb

DAY 265

____ *5-10 minute warm-up*
____ 3 miles on recumbent bike
____ 6 minutes on treadmill
____ 36 floors on stepper
____ 36 jumping jacks
____ 36 push-ups (regular or modified)
____ 3 minutes on recumbent bike
____ 6 minutes on treadmill, incline of "3.5"
____ 36 jump-rope revolutions

DAY 266

____ *5-10 minute warm-up*
____ 4 minutes on treadmill
____ 4 minutes on recumbent bike
____ 4 minutes on elliptical
____ 6 minutes of jump rope (rest when needed)
____ 4 minutes on treadmill
____ 4 minutes on recumbent bike
____ 4 minutes on elliptical
____ 46 push-ups (regular or modified)

"Happiness is when what you think, what you say, and what you do are in harmony."—Mahatma Gandhi

DAY 267

____ *5-10 minute warm-up*
____ 5 minutes on recumbent bike
____ 7 minutes on treadmill, incline of "5"
____ 3 minutes of jumping jacks
____ 4 minutes on treadmill, incline of "3"
____ 6 minutes on upright bike, level "6"
____ 2 minutes of jumping jacks
____ 1 mile on recumbent bike

DAY 268

____ *5-10 minute warm-up*
____ 15 floors on stepper
____ 1.5 miles on upright bike
____ 18 floors on stepper
____ 1.8 miles on upright bike
____ 21 floors on stepper
____ 2.1 miles on upright bike
____ 24 floors on stepper
____ 2.4 miles on upright bike
____ 27 floors on stepper
____ 2.7 miles on upright bike
____ 29 push-ups (regular or modified)
____ 2.9 miles on upright bike

"I used to jog but the ice cubes kept falling out of my glass."—David Lee Roth

DAY 269

____ 5-10 minute warm-up
____ 30 jumping jacks
____ 0.9 mile on treadmill
____ 25 jumping jacks
____ 0.8 mile on treadmill
____ 20 jumping jacks
____ 0.7 mile on treadmill
____ 15 jumping jacks
____ 0.6 mile on treadmill
____ 10 jumping jacks
____ 0.5 mile on treadmill
____ 5 jumping jacks
____ 0.4 mile on treadmill
____ 1 mile on elliptical
____ 0.3 mile on treadmill

DAY 270

____ 5-10 minute warm-up
____ Complete a 5K/10K race or (3.1/6.2 miles) on treadmill

Record your time: _____

"I hated every minute of training, but I said, 'Don't quit. Suffer now and live the rest of your life as a champion.'"—Muhammad Ali

DAY 271
____ *5-10 minute warm-up*
____ 20 push-ups (regular or modified)
____ 1 mile on treadmill
____ 1 mile on upright bike
____ 20 push-ups (regular or modified)
____ 5 minutes on stepper (rest when needed)
____ 1 mile on upright bike
____ 0.5 mile on treadmill
____ 20 floors on stepper
____ 1 mile on upright bike
____ 20 push-ups (regular or modified)

DAY 272
____ *5-10 minute warm-up*
____ 3 minutes on elliptical
____ 5 minutes of jumping jacks
____ 9 minutes on recumbent bike
____ 5 minutes on upright bike
____ 1 mile on elliptical

"Destiny is not a matter of chance; it is a matter of choice. It is not a thing to be waited for; it is a thing to be achieved."—William Jennings Bryan

Day 273

___ *5-10 minute warm-up*
___ 10 floors on stepper
___ 10 push-ups (regular or modified)
___ 5 minutes on treadmill
___ 10 floors on stepper
___ 10 push-ups (regular or modified)
___ 6 minutes on treadmill
___ 10 floors on stepper
___ 10 push-ups (regular or modified)
___ 7 minutes on treadmill, incline of "4"
___ 10 floors on stepper
___ 10 push-ups (regular or modified)
___ 8 minutes on treadmill, incline of "6"
___ 10 floors on stepper
___ 10 push-ups (regular or modified)

Day 274

___ *5-10 minute warm-up*
___ 30 jumping jacks
___ 4 minutes on recumbent bike
___ 3 minutes on Cybex arc trainer
___ 60 jumping jacks
___ 3 minutes on recumbent bike
___ 4 minutes on Cybex arc trainer
___ 90 jumping jacks
___ 7 minutes on recumbent bike
___ 6 minutes on Cybex arc trainer
___ 120 jumping jacks
___ 30 push-ups (regular or modified)

"You don't have to be great to start, but you have to start to be great."—Zig Ziglar

Day 275

____ *5-10 minute warm-up*
____ 1 minute on treadmill (walk)
____ 1 minute on treadmill (jog/run)
____ 15 push-ups (regular or modified)
____ Repeat for 11 minutes

____ 5 minutes on recumbent bike
____ 5 minutes on upright bike
____ 15 push-ups (regular or modified)
____ Rest for 1-2 minutes

____ 1 minute on treadmill (walk)
____ 1 minute on treadmill (jog/run)
____ 15 push-ups (regular or modified)
____ Repeat for 9 minutes

Day 276

____ *5-10 minute warm-up*
____ 1 mile on upright bike
____ 1 mile on recumbent bike
____ 9 minutes on Cybex arc trainer
____ 4 minutes on stepper
____ 7 minutes of jumping jacks (rest when needed)
____ 6 minutes on Cybex arc trainer
____ 9 push-ups (regular or modified)

"If it's important to you, you will find a way. If not, you'll find an excuse."—Anonymous

Day 277

____ *5-10 minute warm-up*
____ 4 minutes on treadmill
____ 4 minutes on upright bike
____ 4 minutes of jump rope (rest when needed)
____ 4 miles on recumbent bike
____ 20 floors on stepper
____ 80 jump-rope revolutions
____ 40 floors on stepper
____ 20 push-ups (regular or modified)

Day 278

____ *5-10 minute warm-up*
____ 5 minutes on elliptical
____ 1 mile on upright bike
____ 1 minute of jumping jacks
____ 8 minutes on elliptical
____ 5 minutes of jumping jacks
____ 8 minutes on upright bike
____ 7 minutes on elliptical, level "8"

"What exactly is success? For me it is to be found not in applause, but in the satisfaction of feeling that one is realizing one's ideal."—Anna Pavlova

Day 279

___ *5-10 minute warm-up*
___ 1 mile on Cybex arc trainer
___ 2 minutes on treadmill, incline of "2"
___ 12 floors on stepper
___ 12 push-ups (regular or modified)
___ Rest 1-2 minutes

___ 1 mile on Cybex arc trainer
___ 4 minutes on treadmill
___ 14 floors on stepper
___ 14 push-ups (regular or modified)

Day 280

___ *5-10 minute warm-up*
___ Fun Workout!*

Aerobics 530	Backpacking 570	Badminton 370
Raking leaves 330	Dancing 450	Basketball 490
Boating 210	Boxing 735	Bowling 245
Canoeing 570	Fishing 250	Frisbee 250
Gardening 330	Golfing 370	Horseback riding 330
Ice skating 570	Mowing lawn 450	Racquetball 570
Soccer 570	Swimming laps 650	Tennis 570
Volleyball 430	Walking (moderate) 300	

Own activity: _____
Duration: _____

*Average calories burned in one hour by a 180-pound person are shown. (http://www.nutristrategy.com/activitylist4.htm)

"I was going to wake up early to go jogging, but my toes voted against me 10 to 1."— Randy Glasbergen

DAY 281

____ *5-10 minute warm-up*
____ 2 minutes on treadmill, incline of "2"
____ 2 minutes on stepper
____ 8 minutes on treadmill, incline of "4"
____ 7 minutes on recumbent bike, level "4"
____ 7 minutes on treadmill, incline of "4"
____ 4 minutes on recumbent bike, level "7"
____ 10 push-ups (regular or modified)

DAY 282

____ *5-10 minute warm-up*
____ 5 minutes on recumbent bike
____ 0.5 mile on Cybex arc trainer
____ 3 minutes of jumping jacks (rest when needed)
____ 5 push-ups (regular or modified)
____ Rest 1-2 minutes

____ 1 mile on Cybex arc trainer
____ 1 minute of jumping jacks
____ 1 mile on recumbent bike
____ 0.5 mile on Cybex arc trainer
____ 50 push-ups (regular or modified)

"The most significant change in a person's life is a change of attitude. Right attitudes produce right actions."—William J. Johnston

DAY 283

____ *5-10 minute warm-up*
____ 10 floors on stepper
____ 1 mile on elliptical, level "10"
____ 1 mile on treadmill, incline of "2.5"
____ 10 push-ups (regular or modified)
____ Rest 1-2 minutes

____ 20 floors on stepper
____ 0.25 mile on elliptical
____ 0.25 mile on treadmill, incline of "5"
____ 20 push-ups (regular or modified)
____ 20 floors on stepper

DAY 284

____ *5-10 minute warm-up*
____ 4 minutes on recumbent bike
____ 40 jump-rope revolutions
____ 4 minutes on Cybex arc trainer
____ 40 jump-rope revolutions
____ Rest 1-2 minutes

____ 80 jump-rope revolutions
____ 8 minutes on Cybex arc trainer
____ 100 jump-rope revolutions
____ 10 minutes on recumbent bike
____ 10 push-ups (regular or modified)
____ 120 jump-rope revolutions
____ 12 minutes on Cybex arc trainer
____ 12 push-ups (regular or modified)

"Wake up with a smile, and go after life…Live it, enjoy it, taste it, smell it, feel it."—Joe Knapp

Day 285
____ 5-10 minute warm-up
____ 8 minutes on treadmill, incline of "2"
____ 28 floors on stepper
____ 5 minutes on treadmill
____ 3 miles on upright bike
____ 82 jumping jacks
____ 8 minutes on treadmill, incline of "2"
____ 28 push-ups (regular or modified)

Day 286
____ 5-10 minute warm-up
____ 3 minutes on elliptical, level "4"
____ 1 mile on recumbent bike, level "4"
____ 4 minutes on elliptical, level "3"
____ 3 miles on recumbent bike, level "3"
____ 4 minutes on elliptical, level "6"
____ 1 mile on recumbent bike, level "6"
____ 6 minutes on elliptical, level "6"
____ 3 minutes on recumbent bike, level "6"

"Dream lofty dreams, and as you dream, so shall you become. Your vision is the promise of what you shall one day be."—James Allen

DAY 287

___ *5-10 minute warm-up*
___ 1 mile on upright bike
___ 100 jump-rope revolutions
___ 1 minute jog/run on treadmill
___ 1 minute walk on treadmill
___ 10 push-ups (regular or modified)
___ Rest 1-2 minutes

___ 100 jump-rope revolutions
___ 1 minute jog/run on treadmill
___ 1 minute walk on treadmill
___ 100 jump-rope revolutions
___ 1 mile on upright bike
___ 10 push-ups (regular or modified)

DAY 288

___ *5-10 minute warm-up*
___ 0.5 mile on Cybex arc trainer
___ 1 mile on upright bike
___ 5 floors on stepper
___ 15 push-ups (regular or modified)
___ 1 mile on upright bike
___ 5 floors on stepper
___ 2 miles on upright bike
___ 10 floors on stepper
___ 10 push-ups (regular or modified)
___ 2 miles on upright bike
___ 10 floors on stepper
___ 0.5 mile on Cybex arc trainer
___ 10 push-ups (regular or modified)

"What counts is not necessarily the size of the dog in the fight—it's the size of the fight in the dog."—Dwight D. Eisenhower

Day 289

___ *5-10 minute warm-up*
___ 6 minutes on upright bike
___ 4 minutes on treadmill
___ 5 minutes on recumbent bike
___ 5 minutes on stepper
___ 5 push-ups (regular or modified)
___ 7 minutes on recumbent bike
___ 3 minutes on treadmill
___ 37 push-ups (regular or modified)

Day 290

___ *5-10 minute warm-up*
___ 1.5 miles on upright bike
___ 15 jumping jacks
___ 15 push-ups (regular or modified)
___ 3 minutes on elliptical, level "3"
___ 33 jumping jacks
___ 15 minutes on elliptical
___ 15 push-ups (regular or modified)
___ 15 jumping jacks
___ 3 miles on upright bike
___ 33 jumping jacks
___ 33 push-ups (regular or modified)

"Joy is what happens to us when we allow ourselves to recognize how good things really are."—Marianne Williamson

Day 291

___ *5-10 minute warm-up*
___ 52 jump-rope revolutions
___ 5 minutes on treadmill, incline of "5.5"
___ 2 miles on upright bike
___ 25 push-ups (regular or modified)
___ 52 jump-rope revolutions
___ 2 miles on upright bike
___ 5 minutes on treadmill, incline of "2"
___ 52 jump-rope revolutions
___ 5 minutes on upright bike
___ 2 minutes on treadmill, incline of "5"

Day 292

___ *5-10 minute warm-up*
___ 0.5 mile on Cybex arc trainer
___ 1 mile on upright bike
___ 9 floors on stepper
___ 9 push-ups (regular or modified)
___ 0.75 mile on Cybex arc trainer
___ 1 mile on upright bike
___ 9 floors on stepper
___ 9 push-ups (regular or modified)
___ 1 mile on Cybex arc trainer
___ 1 mile on upright bike
___ 9 floors on stepper
___ 9 push-ups (regular or modified)

"Motivation is what gets you started. Habit is what keeps you going."
—Jim Ryuh

DAY 293

____ *5-10 minute warm-up*
____ 10 minutes on elliptical
____ 2 minutes of jump rope
____ 2 miles on recumbent bike
____ 4 minutes on elliptical
____ 2 minutes on treadmill
____ 60 jump-rope revolutions
____ 6 minutes on treadmill
____ 6 push-ups (regular or modified)

DAY 294

____ *5-10 minute warm-up*
____ 3 minutes on Cybex arc trainer
____ 7 minutes on upright bike
____ 3 minutes on Cybex arc trainer
____ 7 minutes on recumbent bike
____ 37 push-ups (regular or modified)
____ Rest 1-2 minutes

____ 2 minutes of jumping jacks
____ 2 minutes on stepper
____ 2 minutes of jumping jacks
____ 2 minutes on stepper
____ 2 minutes of jumping jacks
____ 22 push-ups (regular or modified)

"Having a goal is a state of happiness."—E. J. Bartek

Day 295

____ *5-10 minute warm-up*
____ 5 minutes on recumbent bike
____ 4 miles on upright bike
____ 3 minutes of jump rope (rest when needed)
____ 4 minutes on upright bike
____ 3 miles on recumbent bike
____ 3 minutes of jump rope (rest when needed)
____ 33 push-ups (regular or modified)

Day 296

____ *5-10 minute warm-up*
____ 12 floors on stepper
____ 12 push-ups (regular or modified)
____ 1.2 miles on treadmill
____ 12 jump-rope revolutions
____ 12 push-ups (regular or modified)
____ 1.2 miles on upright bike
____ 6 floors on stepper
____ 0.6 mile on treadmill
____ 6 jump-rope revolutions
____ 0.6 mile on treadmill, level "6"

"Do your best every day, and your life will gradually expand into satisfying fullness."—Horatio W. Dresser

DAY 297

____ *5-10 minute warm-up*
____ 1 mile on elliptical
____ 50 jump-rope revolutions
____ 0.5 mile on elliptical
____ 15 push-ups (regular or modified)
____ 50 jump-rope revolutions
____ 0.5 mile on elliptical
____ 15 push-ups (regular or modified)
____ 50 jump-rope revolutions

DAY 298

____ *5-10 minute warm-up*
____ 1 mile on treadmill
____ 3 minutes on recumbent bike
____ 13 push-ups (regular or modified)
____ 0.75 mile on treadmill
____ 3 minutes on upright bike
____ 0.5 mile on treadmill
____ 3 minutes on upright bike
____ 0.25 mile on treadmill
____ 25 push-ups (regular or modified)

"Progress always involves risks. You can't steal second base and keep your foot on first"—Frederick Wilcox

Day 299

___ *5-10 minute warm-up*
___ 1 minute on treadmill (walk)
___ 1 minute on treadmill (jog/run)
___ Repeat for 11 minutes

___ 4 minutes on upright bike
___ 2 miles on recumbent bike
___ 42 push-ups (regular or modified)
___ Rest 1-2 minutes

___ 1 minute on treadmill (walk)
___ 1 minute on treadmill (jog/run)
___ Repeat for 11 minutes

Day 300

___ *5-10 minute warm-up*
___ 300 jumping jacks (rest when needed)
___ 13 minutes on upright bike
___ 13 push-ups (regular or modified)
___ 300 jump-rope revolutions (rest when needed)
___ 3 minutes on Cybex arc trainer
___ 33 push-ups (regular or modified)
___ 300 jumping jacks (rest when needed)

"One filled with joy preaches without preaching."—Mother Teresa

DAY 301

____ *5-10 minute warm-up*
____ Fun Workout!*

Aerobics 530	Backpacking 570	Badminton 370
Raking leaves 330	Dancing 450	Basketball 490
Boating 210	Boxing 735	Bowling 245
Canoeing 570	Fishing 250	Frisbee 250
Gardening 330	Golfing 370	Horseback riding 330
Ice skating 570	Mowing lawn 450	Racquetball 570
Soccer 570	Swimming laps 650	Tennis 570
Volleyball 430	Walking (moderate) 300	

Own activity: _____
Duration: _____

*Average calories burned in one hour by a 180-pound person are shown. (http://www.nutristrategy.com/activitylist4.htm)

DAY 302

____ *5-10 minute warm-up*
____ 2 miles on upright bike
____ 9 minutes on elliptical
____ 29 push-ups (regular or modified)
____ 2 minutes of jumping jacks
____ 2 minutes of jump rope (rest when needed)
____ 22 push-ups (regular or modified)
____ 2 miles on upright bike
____ 9 minutes on elliptical
____ 29 push-ups (regular or modified)

"What a wonderful life I've had! I only wish I'd realized it sooner."
—Colette

DAY 303
___ *5-10 minute warm-up*
___ 2 miles on recumbent bike
___ 6 minutes on stepper
___ 26 push-ups (regular or modified)
___ 1 mile on upright bike
___ 8 minutes on Cybex arc trainer
___ 18 push-ups (regular or modified)
___ 4 minutes on treadmill
___ 7 minutes on stepper
___ 47 push-ups (regular or modified)

DAY 304
___ *5-10 minute warm-up*
___ 4 minutes on Cybex arc trainer
___ 44 jump-rope revolutions
___ 6 minutes on upright bike
___ 66 jump-rope revolutions
___ 4 minutes on upright bike
___ 47 push-ups (regular or modified)
___ 44 jump-rope revolutions
___ 10 minutes on Cybex arc trainer
___ 10 push-ups (regular or modified)
___ 100 jump-rope revolutions

"Your success depends mainly upon what you think of yourself and whether you believe in yourself."—William J. H. Boetcker

DAY 305

____ 5-10 minute warm-up
____ 5 miles on upright bike
____ 6 minutes on treadmill, incline of "5"
____ 5 miles on upright bike
____ 6 minutes on treadmill, incline of "5"
____ 56 push-ups (regular or modified, rest when needed)

DAY 306

____ 5-10 minute warm-up
____ 10 minutes on treadmill
____ 12 minutes on upright bike
____ 12 push-ups (regular or modified)
____ 120 jump-rope revolutions (rest when needed)
____ 120 jumping jacks

*Remember to stay in your Target-Heart-Rate zone.

"Pain is part of being alive, and we need to learn that. Pain does not last forever, nor is it necessarily unbearable, and we need to be taught that."—Rabbi Harold Kushner

DAY 307

____ *5-10 minute warm-up*
____ 2 minutes on stepper
____ 3 minutes on Cybex arc trainer
____ 4 miles on recumbent bike
____ 5 minutes on upright bike
____ 6 minutes on stepper (rest when needed)
____ 70 jump-rope revolutions
____ 80 jumping jacks
____ 90 jump-rope revolutions
____ 10 push-ups (regular or modified)

DAY 308

____ *5-10 minute warm-up*
____ 10 floors on stepper
____ 1 mile on treadmill
____ 10 floors on stepper
____ 0.9 mile on treadmill
____ 10 push-ups (regular or modified)
____ 10 floors on stepper
____ 0.8 mile on treadmill
____ 10 floors on stepper
____ 10 push-ups (regular or modified)
____ 0.7 mile on treadmill
____ 10 floors on stepper
____ 0.6 mile on treadmill
____ 10 floors on stepper
____ 10 push-ups (regular or modified)
____ 0.5 mile on treadmill
____ 10 floors on stepper

"I keep on making what I can't do yet in order to learn to be able to do it."—Pablo Picasso

Day 309

____ *5-10 minute warm-up*
____ 20 floors on stepper
____ 40 jumping jacks
____ 60 floors on stepper
____ 80 jumping jacks
____ 1 mile on recumbent bike, level "8"
____ 2 miles on upright bike
____ 12 push-ups (regular or modified)
____ 100 jumping jacks

Day 310

____ *5-10 minute warm-up*
____ 0.5 mile on treadmill
____ 0.5 mile on upright bike
____ 1 minute on stepper
____ 2 minutes on Cybex arc trainer
____ 3 minutes on stepper
____ 4 minutes on upright bike
____ 5 minutes on Cybex arc trainer
____ 6 minutes on treadmill, incline of "6"
____ 7 minutes on Cybex arc trainer

"Change does not change tradition. It strengthens it. Change is a challenge and an opportunity, not a threat."—Prince Philip, Duke of Edinburgh

Day 311
___ *5-10 minute warm-up*
___ 4 minutes on upright bike
___ 4 minutes on treadmill, incline of "4"
___ 4 miles on recumbent bike
___ 44 push-ups (regular or modified)
___ 4 minutes on treadmill
___ 4 minutes on upright bike

Day 312
___ *5-10 minute warm-up*
___ 5 minutes on Cybex arc trainer
___ 5 minutes on upright bike
___ 15 push-ups (regular or modified)
___ 100 jump-rope revolutions
___ Rest 1-2 minutes

___ 5 minutes on Cybex arc trainer
___ 5 minutes on upright bike
___ 15 push-ups (regular or modified)
___ 100 jump-rope revolutions
___ Rest 1-2 minutes

___ 3 minutes on Cybex arc trainer
___ 3 minutes on treadmill, incline of "3"
___ 100 jump-rope revolutions

"I believe there's an inner power that makes winners or losers. And the winners are the ones who really listen to the truth of their hearts."
—Sylvester Stallone

DAY 313

____ *5-10 minute warm-up*
____ 0.5 mile on treadmill
____ 2 miles on upright bike, level "5"
____ 0.5 mile on treadmill, incline of "5"
____ 25 push-ups (regular or modified)
____ Rest 1-2 minutes

____ 2 miles on upright bike, level "5"
____ 0.5 mile on treadmill, incline of "3"
____ Rest 1-2 minutes

____ 2 miles on upright bike, level "5"
____ 0.5 mile on treadmill
____ 2 miles on upright bike
____ 25 push-ups (regular or modified)

DAY 314

____ *5-10 minute warm-up*
____ 2 miles on recumbent bike
____ 2 minutes on stepper
____ 2 minutes of jumping jacks
____ 22 push-ups (regular or modified)
____ 4 miles on recumbent bike
____ 4 minutes on stepper
____ 4 minutes of jumping jacks (rest when needed)
____ 4 minute walk/jog on treadmill
____ 22 push-ups (regular or modified)

"Whether you think you can, or you think you can't—you're right."
—Henry Ford

DAY 315
___ *5-10 minute warm-up*
___ Complete a 5K/10K race or (3.1/6.2 miles) on treadmill

Record your time: _____

DAY 316
___ *5-10 minute warm-up*
___ 0.5 mile on Cybex arc trainer
___ 3.5 miles on upright bike
___ 35 push-ups (regular or modified)
___ 0.5 mile on elliptical
___ 0.5 mile on Cybex arc trainer
___ 3.5 miles on upright bike
___ 35 push-ups (regular or modified)
___ 0.5 mile on elliptical
___ 0.5 mile on Cybex arc trainer

"Continuity gives us roots; change gives us branches, letting us stretch and grow and reach heights."—Pauline R. Kezer

Day 317

____ *5-10 minute warm-up*
____ 7 floors on stepper
____ 70 jump-rope revolutions
____ 7 minutes on treadmill, incline of "7"
____ 17 push-ups (regular or modified)
____ Rest 1-2 minutes

____ 7 floors on stepper
____ 70 jump-rope revolutions
____ 7 minutes on treadmill, incline of "7"
____ 7 minutes on upright bike, level "7"
____ 17 push-ups (regular or modified)
____ 0.75 mile on treadmill

Day 318

____ *5-10 minute warm-up*
____ 3 miles on upright bike
____ 1.3 miles on Cybex arc trainer
____ 13 push-ups (regular or modified)
____ 3 miles on upright bike
____ 0.3 mile on Cybex arc trainer
____ 30 jumping jacks
____ 3 minutes on upright bike
____ 13 push-ups (regular or modified)

"Progress is impossible without change, and those who cannot change their minds cannot change anything."—Attributed to George Bernard Shaw

DAY 319

____ *5-10 minute warm-up*
____ 2 miles on upright bike
____ 10 floors on stepper
____ 10 push-ups (regular or modified)
____ 20 jumping jacks
____ 10 minutes on elliptical
____ 2 miles on upright bike
____ 10 minutes on elliptical
____ 10 push-ups (regular or modified)

DAY 320

____ *5-10 minute warm-up*
____ Fun Workout!*

Aerobics 530	Backpacking 570	Badminton 370
Raking leaves 330	Dancing 450	Basketball 490
Boating 210	Boxing 735	Bowling 245
Canoeing 570	Fishing 250	Frisbee 250
Gardening 330	Golfing 370	Horseback riding 330
Ice skating 570	Mowing lawn 450	Racquetball 570
Soccer 570	Swimming laps 650	Tennis 570
Volleyball 430	Walking (moderate) 300	

Own activity: _____
Duration: _____

*Average calories burned in one hour by a 180-pound person are shown. (http://www.nutristrategy.com/activitylist4.htm)

"You have to believe in happiness, or happiness never comes."—
Douglas Malloch

DAY 321

____ *5-10 minute warm-up*
____ 5 minutes on treadmill, incline of "3"
____ 3 minutes on treadmill, incline of "5"
____ 3 minutes on Cybex arc trainer
____ 3 minutes of jump-rope revolutions (rest when needed)
____ 2 miles on upright bike
____ 1 mile on Cybex arc trainer

DAY 322

____ *5-10 minute warm-up*
____ 4 minutes on treadmill, incline of "6"
____ 4 minutes on elliptical, level "6"
____ 5 minutes on treadmill
____ 4 minutes of jump rope (rest when needed)
____ 6 minutes on elliptical, level "6"
____ 3 miles on recumbent bike, level "6"

"Where focus goes, energy flows. And if you don't take the time to focus on what matters, then you're living a life of someone else's design."—Tony Robbins

DAY 323

____ *5-10 minute warm-up*
____ 4 minutes on Cybex arc trainer
____ 8 floors on stepper
____ 8 push-ups (regular or modified)
____ 4 minutes on upright bike
____ 8 floors on stepper
____ 8 push-ups (regular or modified)
____ 4 minutes on Cybex arc trainer
____ 8 floors on stepper
____ 8 push-ups (regular or modified)
____ Rest 1-2 minutes

____ 2 minutes on Cybex arc trainer
____ 4 floors on stepper
____ 2 minutes on upright bike
____ 4 floors on stepper
____ 2 minutes on Cybex arc trainer
____ 4 floors on stepper
____ 2 minutes on recumbent bike

DAY 324

____ *5-10 minute warm-up*
____ 4 minutes on treadmill
____ 7 minutes on upright bike
____ 11 minutes on elliptical
____ 11 push-ups (regular or modified)
____ 100 jump-rope revolutions
____ 4 minutes on treadmill
____ 1 mile on recumbent bike

"Hard work pays off in the future. Laziness pays off now."—Steven Wright

DAY 325

____ *5-10 minute warm-up*
____ 1 minute on treadmill (walk)
____ 1 minute on treadmill (jog/run)
____ Repeat for 16 minutes

____ 3 minutes on upright bike
____ 3 miles on recumbent bike
____ 33 push-ups (regular or modified)
____ Rest 1-2 minutes

____ 1 minute on treadmill (walk)
____ 1 minute on treadmill (jog/run)
____ Repeat for 8 minutes

DAY 326

____ *5-10 minute warm-up*
____ 4 minutes on upright bike
____ 6 minutes on treadmill
____ 16 push-ups (regular or modified)
____ 5 minutes on recumbent bike
____ 8 floors on stepper
____ 2 miles on upright bike
____ 12 push-ups (regular or modified)
____ 7 minutes on upright bike
____ 3 minutes on stepper

"Let today be the day you love yourself enough to no longer just dream about a better life; let it be the day you act upon it."—Steve Maraboli

DAY 327
___ *5-10 minute warm-up*
___ 0.5 mile on upright bike
___ 0.5 mile on elliptical
___ 1 mile on recumbent bike
___ 1 mile on upright bike, level "7"
___ 15 push-ups (regular or modified)
___ 1.5 miles on elliptical
___ 1.5 miles on recumbent bike
___ 15 push-ups (regular or modified)
___ 3 miles on upright bike

DAY 328
___ *5-10 minute warm-up*
___ 28 floors on stepper
___ 2.8 miles on upright bike
___ 0.8 mile on Cybex arc trainer
___ 18 floors on stepper
___ 18 push-ups (regular or modified)
___ 1.4 miles on upright bike
___ 0.4 mile on Cybex arc trainer
___ 8 floors on stepper
___ 8 push-ups (regular or modified)

"The three Cs of life: choices, chances, and changes. You must make a choice to take a chance or your life will never change."—Anonymous

Day 329

____ *5-10 minute warm-up*
____ 4 minutes on treadmill, incline of "2"
____ 1 minute on treadmill, incline of "7"
____ 3 minutes on treadmill, incline of "3"
____ 1 mile on upright bike
____ 1 mile on recumbent bike, level "2"
____ 13 push-ups (regular or modified)
____ Rest 1-2 minutes

____ 4 minutes on treadmill, incline of "2"
____ 1 minute on treadmill, incline of "7"
____ 3 minutes on treadmill, incline of "3"
____ 1 mile on upright bike
____ 1 mile on recumbent bike, level "2"
____ 11 push-ups (regular or modified)

Day 330

____ *5-10 minute warm-up*
____ 10 minutes on elliptical
____ 10 push-ups (regular or modified)
____ 8 minutes on stepper
____ 6 minutes on recumbent bike
____ 6 push-ups (regular or modified)
____ 4 minutes on Cybex arc trainer
____ 2 miles on upright bike

"Security is mostly a superstition. It does not exist in nature...Life is either a daring adventure or nothing."—Helen Keller

DAY 331
___ *5-10 minute warm-up*
___ 3 minutes on upright bike
___ 9 minutes on elliptical
___ 2 minutes of jump rope (rest when needed)
___ 5 minutes on elliptical
___ 4 minutes of jump rope (rest when needed)
___ 7 minutes on elliptical

DAY 332
___ *5-10 minute warm-up*
___ 0.85 mile on treadmill
___ 3 minutes on recumbent bike
___ 0.75 mile on treadmill
___ 3 minutes on recumbent bike
___ 0.65 mile on treadmill
___ 3 minutes on recumbent bike
___ 0.55 mile on treadmill
___ 3 minutes on recumbent bike
___ 0.45 mile on treadmill
___ 3 minutes on recumbent bike
___ 0.35 mile on treadmill
___ 35 push-ups (regular or modified)

"Being happy doesn't mean everything is perfect. It means you've decided to look beyond the imperfections."—Anonymous

DAY 333

____ *5-10 minute warm-up*
____ 76 jumping jacks
____ 6 minutes on upright bike
____ 0.76 mile on elliptical
____ 4 minutes on Cybex arc trainer
____ 7 minutes on upright bike
____ 47 push-ups (regular or modified)
____ 0.76 mile on elliptical
____ 76 jumping jacks

DAY 334

____ *5-10 minute warm-up*
____ 8 floors on stepper
____ 5 minutes on treadmill, incline of "8"
____ 8 minutes on stepper
____ 5 minutes on treadmill
____ 8 miles on upright bike
____ 58 push-ups (regular or modified)

"We tend to forget that happiness doesn't come as a result of getting something we don't have, but rather of recognizing and appreciating what we do have."—Frederick Koenig

Day 335

____ *5-10 minute warm-up*
____ 1 minute of jumping jacks
____ 1 mile on recumbent bike
____ 1 minute of jumping jacks
____ Rest 1-2 minutes

____ 9 minutes on upright bike
____ 9 push-ups (regular or modified)
____ 9 floors on stepper
____ 9 push-ups (regular or modified)
____ 9 minutes on Cybex arc trainer
____ Rest 1-2 minutes

____ 1 minute of jumping jacks
____ 1 mile on recumbent bike
____ 1 minute of jumping jacks

Day 336

____ *5-10 minute warm-up*
____ 1 mile on upright bike
____ 1 mile on elliptical
____ 11 push-ups (regular or modified)
____ 3 minutes on upright bike, level "7"
____ 4 minutes on elliptical, level "7"
____ 2 miles on upright bike, level "2"
____ 9 minutes on elliptical, level "2"
____ 29 push-ups (regular or modified)

"Those who think they have no time for healthy eating will sooner or later have to find time for illness."—Attributed to Edward Stanley

DAY 337

___ *5-10 minute warm-up*
___ 12 minutes on treadmill
___ 34 floors on stepper
___ 56 jump-rope revolutions
___ 78 jumping jacks
___ 91 jump-rope revolutions
___ 10 minutes on treadmill
___ 10 push-ups (regular or modified)

DAY 338

___ *5-10 minute warm-up*
___ 3 minutes on upright bike
___ 7 floors on stepper
___ 4 minutes on Cybex arc trainer
___ 9 minutes on upright bike
___ 1 mile on Cybex arc trainer
___ 10 floors on stepper
___ 3 minutes on upright bike

"To seek one's goal and to drive toward it, stealing one's heart, is most uplifting."—Henrik Ibsen

DAY 339

____ 5-10 minute warm-up
____ 2.6 miles on recumbent bike, level "2"
____ 25 push-ups (regular or modified)
____ 2.4 miles on upright bike, level "2"
____ 23 jumping jacks
____ 22 push-ups (regular or modified)
____ 21 jump-rope revolutions
____ 2.0 miles on upright bike
____ 19 jumping jacks
____ 1.8 miles on treadmill

DAY 340

____ 5-10 minute warm-up
____ Fun Workout!*

Aerobics 530	Backpacking 570	Badminton 370
Raking leaves 330	Dancing 450	Basketball 490
Boating 210	Boxing 735	Bowling 245
Canoeing 570	Fishing 250	Frisbee 250
Gardening 330	Golfing 370	Horseback riding 330
Ice skating 570	Mowing lawn 450	Racquetball 570
Soccer 570	Swimming laps 650	Tennis 570
Volleyball 430	Walking (moderate) 300	

Own activity: _____

Duration: _____

*Average calories burned in one hour by a 180-pound person are shown. (http://www.nutristrategy.com/activitylist4.htm)

"There are three ingredients in the good life: learning, earning, and yearning."—Christopher Morley

DAY 341
____ 5-10 minute warm-up
____ 4 minutes on Cybex arc trainer
____ 4 minutes on stepper
____ 1 mile on Cybex arc trainer
____ 1 minute on stepper
____ 11 push-ups (regular or modified)
____ Rest 1-2 minutes

____ 4 minutes on upright bike, level "4"
____ 4 minutes on stepper (rest when needed)
____ 1 mile on upright bike, level "10"
____ 1 mile on upright bike, level "4"
____ 11 push-ups (regular or modified)

DAY 342
____ 5-10 minute warm-up
____ 4 minutes on treadmill, incline of "2"
____ 2 minutes on treadmill, incline of "4"
____ 6 minutes on elliptical
____ 3 miles on recumbent bike
____ 5 minutes on treadmill, incline of "5"
____ 35 push-ups (regular or modified)

"Minutes are worth more than money. Spend them wisely."—Thomas P. Murphy

Day 343

____ *5-10 minute warm-up*
____ 1 mile on Cybex arc trainer
____ 2 miles on upright bike
____ 3 minutes of jump rope (rest when needed)
____ 4 floors on stepper
____ 1 mile on upright bike
____ 2 minutes of jump rope (rest when needed)
____ 3 minutes on Cybex arc trainer
____ 4 minutes on recumbent bike
____ 34 push-ups (regular or modified)

Day 344

____ *5-10 minute warm-up*
____ 70 jumping jacks
____ 3 minutes on stepper
____ 3 minutes on treadmill, incline of "3"
____ 70 jumping jacks
____ 6 minutes on recumbent bike
____ 8 floors on stepper
____ 8 push-ups (regular or modified)
____ 70 jumping jacks
____ 4 minutes on treadmill, incline of "8"
____ 2 miles on recumbent bike
____ 70 jumping jacks

"The possibilities are unlimited as long as you are true to your life's purpose."—Marcia Wieder

Day 345

___ *5-10 minute warm-up*
___ 0.5 mile on elliptical
___ 10 floors on stepper
___ 1.5 miles on upright bike
___ 2 miles on upright bike
___ 25 floors on stepper
___ 25 push-ups (regular or modified)
___ 3 minutes on elliptical
___ 3.5 miles on upright bike
___ 4 minutes on stepper
___ 4.5 miles on upright bike

Day 346

___ *5-10 minute warm-up*
___ 9 minutes on treadmill
___ 99 jumping jacks
___ 7 minutes on treadmill
___ 77 jumping jacks
___ 5 minutes on recumbent bike
___ 55 jumping jacks
___ 3 minutes on treadmill
___ 33 jumping jacks
___ 1 mile on upright bike
___ 11 push-ups (regular or modified)

"As soon as you trust yourself, you will know how to live."—Johann Wolfgang von Goethe

DAY 347

____ *5-10 minute warm-up*
____ 2.5 miles on upright bike
____ 1 mile on Cybex arc trainer
____ 15 floors on stepper
____ 15 push-ups (regular or modified)
____ 2 miles on upright bike
____ 0.75 mile on Cybex arc trainer
____ 17 floors on stepper
____ 17 push-ups (regular or modified)

DAY 348

____ *5-10 minute warm-up*
____ 6 minutes on treadmill, incline of "6"
____ 66 jump-rope revolutions
____ 10 minutes on elliptical
____ 10 push-ups (regular or modified)
____ 100 jump-rope revolutions (rest when needed)
____ 8 minutes on treadmill
____ 88 jump-rope revolutions
____ 1 mile on recumbent bike

"Believe that your life is worth living, and your belief will help create that fact."—William James

Day 349
____ *5-10 minute warm-up*
____ 1 mile on elliptical
____ 3 miles on upright bike
____ 13 push-ups (regular or modified)
____ 0.75 mile on elliptical
____ 2 miles on upright bike
____ 1 mile on recumbent bike
____ 12 push-ups (regular or modified)

Day 350
____ *5-10 minute warm-up*
____ 1 minute on treadmill (walk)
____ 1 minute on treadmill (jog/run)
____ Repeat for 10 minutes

____ 3 miles on recumbent bike
____ 3 minutes on upright bike
____ 33 push-ups (regular or modified)
____ Rest 1-2 minutes

____ 1 minute on treadmill (walk)
____ 1 minute on treadmill (jog/run)
____ Repeat for 15 minutes

"Exercise to stimulate, not to annihilate. The world wasn't formed in a day, and neither were we. Set small goals and build upon them."—Lee Haney

DAY 351

____ *5-10 minute warm-up*
____ 14 floors on stepper
____ 1.4 miles on Cybex arc trainer
____ 14 push-ups (regular or modified)
____ 15 floors on stepper
____ 1.5 miles on Cybex arc trainer
____ 15 push-ups (regular or modified)

DAY 352

____ *5-10 minute warm-up*
____ 6 minutes on treadmill, incline of "3"
____ 15 minutes on upright bike
____ 3 miles on recumbent bike, level "3"
____ 6 minutes on treadmill, incline of "3"
____ 15 push-ups (regular or modified)

*Remember to stay in your Target-Heart-Rate zone.

"My idea of exercise is a good brisk sit."—Phyllis Diller

Day 353

___ *5-10 minute warm-up*
___ 6 minutes on recumbent bike, level "6"
___ 6 minutes on stepper
___ 6 minutes on elliptical, level "8"
___ 4 minutes on recumbent bike
___ 4 minutes on elliptical, level "4"
___ 4 minutes on stepper
___ 44 push-ups (regular or modified)

Day 354

___ *5-10 minute warm-up*
___ 50 jumping jacks
___ 1 mile on treadmill
___ 50 jumping jacks
___ 1 mile on Cybex arc trainer
___ 0.5 mile on treadmill
___ 50 jumping jacks
___ 0.5 mile on Cybex arc trainer
___ 50 jumping jacks

"We don't stop playing because we grow old; we grow old because we stop playing."—George Bernard Shaw

Day 355

___ *5-10 minute warm-up*
___ 2 miles on upright bike
___ 2 miles on recumbent bike
___ 6 minutes on elliptical
___ 22 push-ups (regular or modified)
___ 2 miles on upright bike
___ 2 miles on recumbent bike
___ 6 minutes on elliptical

Day 356

___ *5-10 minute warm-up*
___ 18 floors on stepper
___ 18 push-ups (regular or modified)
___ 8 minutes on Cybex arc trainer
___ 8 minutes on upright bike, level "8"
___ 22 floors on stepper
___ 12 minutes on Cybex arc trainer
___ 12 push-ups (regular or modified)

"The secret of discipline is motivation. When a man is sufficiently moti-
vated, discipline will take care of itself."—Sir Alexander Paterson

DAY 357

___ *5-10 minute warm-up*
___ 0.8 mile on treadmill
___ 25 jumping jacks
___ 25 push-ups (regular or modified)
___ 1.8 miles on elliptical
___ 100 jumping jacks
___ 0.4 mile on treadmill
___ 25 jumping jacks
___ 25 push-ups (regular or modified)
___ 0.6 mile on elliptical

DAY 358

___ *5-10 minute warm-up*
___ 30 floors on stepper
___ 3 miles on recumbent bike
___ 20 floors on stepper
___ 6 minutes on recumbent bike
___ 3 miles on upright bike
___ 10 floors on stepper
___ 2 miles on recumbent bike
___ 1 mile on upright bike
___ 30 push-ups (regular or modified)

"The pleasure which we most rarely experience gives us greatest delight."—Epictetus

Day 359

____ *5-10 minute warm-up*

____Complete a 5K/10K race or (3.1/6.2 miles) on treadmill

Record your time: _____

Day 360

____ *5-10 minute warm-up*

____ Fun Workout!*

Aerobics 530	Backpacking 570	Badminton 370
Raking leaves 330	Dancing 450	Basketball 490
Boating 210	Boxing 735	Bowling 245
Canoeing 570	Fishing 250	Frisbee 250
Gardening 330	Golfing 370	Horseback riding 330
Ice skating 570	Mowing lawn 450	Racquetball 570
Soccer 570	Swimming laps 650	Tennis 570
Volleyball 430	Walking (moderate) 300	

Own activity: _____

Duration: _____

*Average calories burned in one hour by a 180-pound person are shown. (http://www.nutristrategy.com/activitylist4.htm)

"Happiness is nothing more than good health and a bad memory."
—Albert Schweitzer

Day 361

___ *5-10 minute warm-up*
___ 11 minutes on treadmill
___ 9 minutes on upright bike
___ 7 minutes on elliptical
___ 5 minutes on treadmill, incline of "5"
___ 11 push-ups (regular or modified)

Day 362

___ *5-10 minute warm-up*
___ 40 jump-rope revolutions
___ 1 mile on Cybex arc trainer
___ 50 jump-rope revolutions
___ 1 mile on upright bike
___ 60 jump-rope revolutions
___ 1 mile on Cybex arc trainer
___ 70 jump-rope revolutions
___ 1 mile on upright bike
___ 80 jump-rope revolutions
___ 1 mile on upright bike
___ 90 push-ups (regular or modified, rest when needed)

"You'll see it when you believe it."—Wayne Dyer

Day 363

____ *5-10 minute warm-up*
____ 2 miles on recumbent bike
____ 6 miles on upright bike
____ 2 miles on recumbent bike
____ 26 push-ups (regular or modified)
____ 1 mile on recumbent bike
____ 5 miles on upright bike
____ 1 mile on recumbent bike
____ 15 push-ups (regular or modified)

Day 364

____ *5-10 minute warm-up*
____ 12 floors on stepper
____ 12 minutes on treadmill
____ 12 push-ups (regular or modified)
____ 8 minutes on elliptical
____ 8 minutes on treadmill
____ 12 floors on stepper
____ 12 jumping jacks
____ 12 push-ups (regular or modified)

"Don't stop when you're tired, stop when you're done."—Manuel Tratter

DAY 365

____ *5-10 minute warm-up*

____ 365 jump-rope revolutions (rest when needed)

____ 3 miles on recumbent bike

____ 6 minutes on treadmill

____ 5 minutes on upright bike

____ 365 jump-rope revolutions (rest when needed)

DAY 366 (EVERY FOUR YEARS)

____ Relax, Get a Massage, Eat Healthy, and Do Nothing Else!

"Happiness is something that comes into our lives through doors we don't even remember leaving open."—Rose Wilder Lane

Thank you for opening this door, and congratulations on completing 365 days of cardio fitness! My hope is that you were able to go to places you never could imagine, accomplish the unthinkable, and, in the process, change your health forever.

Next steps: recycle, reuse and/or repeat the workouts in this book.

This book was written to be used multiple times and the workouts can be completed in any order.

So mix it up, have fun and grab a partner to share the journey!

When you don't give up, you cannot fail.

Visit me and share your success story on my website at www.365customcardio.com